RENAL
PHYSIOLOGY

RENAL PHYSIOLOGY

Third Edition

Arthur J. Vander, M.D.
Professor of Physiology
University of Michigan

McGraw-Hill Book Company

New York St. Louis San Francisco Auckland Bogotá Guatemala Hamburg
Johannesburg Lisbon London Madrid Mexico Montreal New Delhi Panama
Paris San Juan São Paulo Singapore Sydney Tokyo Toronto

RENAL PHYSIOLOGY

Copyright © 1985, 1980, 1975 by McGraw-Hill, Inc. All rights reserved. Printed in the United States of America. Except as permitted under the United States Copyright Act of 1976, no part of this publication may be reproduced or distributed in any form or by any means, or stored in a data base or retrieval system, without the prior written permission of the publisher.

1 2 3 4 5 6 7 8 9 0 DOC DOC 8 9 8 7 6 5

This book was set in Times New Roman by McGraw-Hill Information Systems and Technology; the editor was Beth Ann Kaufman; the production supervisor was Thomas J. LoPinto. The cover was designed by Edward R. Schultheis. Project supervision was done by The Total Book.
R. R. Donnelley & Sons Company was printer and binder.

ISBN 0-07-066959-7

Library of Congress Cataloging in Publication Data

Vander, Arthur J   date
   Renal physiology.

   Bibliography: p.
   Includes index.
   1. Kidneys. I. Title. [DNLM: 1. Kidney—Physiology.
WJ300.3 V228r]
QP249.V36 1985   612'.463   84-14427
ISBN 0-07-066959-7

CONTENTS

PREFACE

This book is my attempt to identify the essential core content of renal physiology appropriate for medical students and to present it in a way which permits the student to master the material independently, i.e., with no (or very few) accompanying lectures by the instructor. I have been gratified by the wide use the first two editions have achieved and the many letters I have received from medical students (and clinicians) who found they were, indeed, able to master its contents by independent study.

Accordingly, my major goals in preparing this third edition have been to update the material thoroughly and to strive for greater clarity of exposition (to this latter end, a large number of new flow diagrams has been added, others deleted, and still others changed), but not to alter the level of coverage, except where new information has required it. For example, I have significantly expanded the coverage of glomerular-filtration dynamics, mechanisms of sodium and chloride reabsorption, tubular handling of potassium, and nephron heterogeneity. The task of sticking to my intent of presenting only what I consider core material was even more painful this time because of the explosion of information in renal physiology over the past 4 years.

My selection of this core material is made explicit in a comprehensive list of behavioral objectives, which tell students specifically what I believe they should know and be able to do by the book's completion. Obviously, no two instructors would come up with exactly the same core material, but it is a simple matter for instructors to give students a supplementary list of goals to be added or deleted. The information required to achieve any additional goals not covered in the book would, of course, have to be provided by other reading assignments or lectures. However, my belief, based on consultations with other physiologists and clinicians, is that these discrepancies are likely to be few. Of much greater importance is the fact that the behavioral goals (in essence, the content of the book) are explicitly defined so that any such differences are easily determined. This also makes the book quite usable for students in other health sciences, whose required core of information might differ from that of medical students.

In addition to the comprehensive objectives, I have included a large number of study questions considerably expanded for this edition with annotated answers. Unlike the lists of objectives, the study questions are neither systematic nor comprehensive in their coverage. Rather, they generally deal with areas I found usually difficult for students and give them practice and additional feedback.

I advise the student to go through the book one chapter at a time. Some students profit by using the objectives to guide their readings as they proceed through a chapter. In any case, at the end of each chapter go over the objectives in detail and the study questions (at the back of the book) relevant to the chapter. They provide you with the means for determining whether you have mastered the material and for identifying those specific areas which require more work.

I should like to point out several characteristics of the book common to most texts but particularly common in this type of book. I have rarely included the original research upon which this core of knowledge rests, nor have I been able to explore the fascinating controversies in virtually every area. Therefore, the Suggested Readings at the back of the book have been expanded and are of considerable importance for the student who wishes to pursue any subject in greater depth. They are almost all review articles, and their bibliographies provide an entry into the original research literature.

The question of how to handle complexity and controversy in such a book is a particularly perplexing one. First, it has gotten to the point where almost every statement of "fact" in renal physiology often requires qualification. Second, and related to this, is the multiplicity of processes and controls for specific phenomena (such as sodium reabsorption, for example). Accordingly, I have often used the terms "major" or "most important" in describing those processes included in the book, and either simply ignored some of the others altogether or included them in footnotes. Footnotes have also been used for citing opposing views in certain particularly important controversies. (For these reasons, the number of footnotes in the book has increased, but my advice to most students is to ignore the footnotes completely.) Obviously, such decisions are always arbitrary, to a large degree, and I can only apologize, in advance, to those of my colleagues who feel I have slighted their work.

Also, for those colleagues who delight (as I do) in checking out how much a new edition has been enlarged, I would like to stress that much of the modest increase in size of this edition, compared to the last, represents additional clarifying flow-diagrams, study questions, and suggested readings.

Finally, I should like once again to thank Peggy Rogers for her splendid typing of the manuscript.

Arthur J. Vander

RENAL PHYSIOLOGY

CHAPTER 1

FUNCTION AND STRUCTURE OF THE KIDNEYS

OBJECTIVES

The student states the balance concept.

The student knows the functions of the kidneys.
1 Lists seven functions
2 States the major components of the renin-angiotensin system and their biochemical interrelations
3 Defines inactive renin, extrarenal renin, and angiotensin III
4 States the role of erythropoietin

The student defines important gross structures and knows their interrelationships: renal pelvis, calyxes, renal pyramids, medulla (inner and outer), cortex, papilla

The student understands the interrelationships between the components of a nephron.
1 Defines glomerulus and tubule
2 Draws the relationship between glomerular capillaries, Bowman's capsule, and the proximal tubule
3 States the three layers separating the lumen of the glomerular capillaries and Bowman's space; defines podocytes, foot processes, slits, and slit diaphragms
4 Defines glomerular mesangium and states its functions
5 Lists in order the individual tubular segments; defines proximal tubule, loop of Henle, distal tubule, and collecting duct

6 Describes the differences between superficial cortical, midcortical, and juxtamedullary nephrons
7 Defines interstitial cells
8 Defines juxtaglomerular apparatus and describes its three cell types; states the function of the granular cells
9 Describes, in general terms, the renal prostaglandins and the renal kallikrein-kinin system

The student understands the blood supply to the nephron.
1 Lists, in order, the vessels through which blood flows from renal artery to renal vein
2 Defines vasa recta and vascular bundles

FUNCTIONS

Regulation of Water and Electrolyte Balance

A cell's function depends not only upon receiving a continuous supply of nutrients and eliminating its metabolic end products but also upon the existence of stable physicochemical conditions in the extracellular fluid bathing it, Claude Bernard's "internal environment." Maintenance of this stability is the primary function of the kidneys.

Since the extracellular fluid occupies an intermediate position between the external environment and the cells, the concentration of any substance within it can be altered by exchange in either direction. Exchanges with cells are called *internal exchanges*. For example, a decrease in extracellular potassium concentration is followed by a counteracting movement of potassium out of cells into the extracellular fluid. Each type of ion is stored in cells or in bone in significant amounts, which can be partially depleted or expanded without damage to the storage site. But these stores are limited, and in the long run any deficit or excess of total body water or total body electrolyte must be compensated by exchanges with the external environment, i.e., by changes in intake or output.

A substance appears in the body either as a result of ingestion or as a product of metabolism. Conversely, a substance can be excreted from the body or consumed in a metabolic reaction. Therefore, if the quantity of any substance in the body is to be maintained at a constant level over a period of time, the total amounts ingested and produced must equal the total amounts excreted and consumed. This is a general statement of the *balance concept*. For water and hydrogen ion all four possible pathways apply. However, balance is simpler for the mineral electrolytes. Since they are neither synthesized nor consumed by cells, their total body balance reflects only ingestion versus excretion.

As an example, let us describe the balance for total body water (Table 1-1). It should be recognized that these are average values, which are subject

Table 1-1 Normal Routes of Water Gain and Loss in Adults

Route	mL/day
Intake	
Drunk	1200
In food	1000
Metabolically produced	350
Total	2550
Output	
Insensible loss (skin and lungs)	900
Sweat	50
In feces	100
Urine	1500
Total	2550

to considerable variation. The two sources of body water are metabolically produced water, resulting largely from the oxidation of carbohydrates, and ingested water, obtained from liquids and so-called solid food (a rare steak is approximately 70 percent water).

There are four sites from which water is lost to the external environment: skin, lungs, gastrointestinal tract, and kidneys. The loss of water by evaporation from the cells of the skin and the lining of respiratory passageways is a continuous process, often referred to as *insensible loss* because the person is unaware of its occurrence. Additional water can be made available for evaporation from the skin by the production of sweat.

Under normal conditions, as can be seen from the table, water loss exactly equals water gain, and no net change of body water occurs. This is obviously no accident but the result of precise regulatory mechanisms. The question then is: Which processes involved in water balance are controlled to make the gains and losses balance? The answer, as we shall see, is voluntary intake (*thirst*) and urinary loss. This does not mean that none of the other processes is controlled, but it does mean their control is not primarily oriented toward water balance. Carbohydrate catabolism, the major source of water from oxidation, is controlled by mechanisms directed toward regulation of energy balance. Sweat production is controlled by mechanisms directed toward temperature regulation. Insensible loss in humans is truly uncontrolled. Fecal water loss is generally unchanging and is normally quite small (but can be severe in vomiting or diarrhea).

The mechanism of thirst is certainly of great importance, since body deficits of water, regardless of cause, must be made up by ingestion of water. But it is also true that our fluid intake is often influenced more by habit and by sociological factors than by the need to regulate body water.

The control of urinary water loss is the major automatic mechanism by which body water is regulated.

By similar analyses, we find that the body balances of many of the ions determining the properties of the extracellular fluid are regulated primarily by the kidneys. To appreciate the importance of these kidney regulations one need only make a partial list of the more important simple inorganic substances in the internal environment that are regulated in large part by the kidneys: water, sodium, potassium, chloride, calcium, magnesium, sulfate, phosphate, and hydrogen ion. However, the kidneys are not the major regulators of all essential inorganic substances; in particular, the body balances of many of the trace elements, such as zinc and iron, are regulated mainly by control of gastrointestinal absorption of the element or by control of biliary secretion rather than by renal excretion. This is, in large part, also true of calcium. Nevertheless, even for these elements some renal excretion occurs and may constitute an important source of bodily imbalance in various diseases. Finally, the kidneys also take part in the regulation of organic nutrients; this will be discussed in subsequent chapters.

Excretion of Metabolic Waste Products

The regulatory role just described is obviously quite different from the popular conception of the kidneys as glorified garbage disposal units which rid the body of assorted wastes and poisons. It is true that some of the chemical reactions which occur within cells result ultimately in end products that must be eliminated. These end products are called waste products because they serve no known biological function in humans. For example, the catabolism of protein produces approximately 30 g of urea per day. Other end products produced in relatively large quantities are uric acid (from nucleic acids), creatinine (from muscle creatine), bilirubin and other end products of hemoglobin breakdown, and the metabolites of various hormones. There are many others, not all of which have been completely identified. Most of these substances are eliminated from the body as rapidly as they are produced, primarily by way of the kidneys. Some of them, e.g., urea, are relatively harmless, but the accumulation of others within the body during periods of renal malfunction accounts for some of the disordered body functions in the patient suffering from severe kidney disease. We still are not sure as to the identity of these "toxins" or which of the problems occurring in renal disease are due to them, rather than to disordered water-and-electrolyte metabolism.

Excretion of Foreign Chemicals

The kidneys have another general excretory function, the elimination from the body of many foreign chemicals, such as drugs, pesticides, food additives, and their metabolites.

Regulation of Arterial Blood Pressure

The kidneys are intimately involved in the regulation of arterial blood pressure by several mechanisms. First, sodium balance is a critical determinant of cardiac output (and, possibly, arteriolar resistance, over any long time period), and the kidneys, as stated above, regulate this balance. Second, the kidneys function as endocrine glands in the *renin-angiotensin system,* a hormonal complex of enzymes, proteins, and peptides that are important in the regulation of arterial pressure.

The Renin-angiotensin System   Renin is a proteolytic enzyme secreted into the blood by the kidneys, specifically by the granular cells of the juxtaglomerular apparatuses (see below). Once in the bloodstream, renin catalyzes the splitting of a decapeptide, *angiotensin I,* from a plasma protein known as *angiotensinogen,* which is secreted by the liver and is always present in the plasma in high concentration. Under the influence of another enzyme, *angiotensin-converting enzyme,* the terminal two amino acids are then split from the relatively inactive angiotensin I to yield the highly active octapeptide *angiotensin II.* Some converting enzyme is present in plasma but most is on the endothelial surface of blood vessels, particularly the pulmonary capillaries; accordingly, the conversion of angiotensin I to angiotensin II occurs mainly as blood flows through the lungs.

Thus, angiotensin II is a hormone in that it reaches its target organs (including the kidneys, as we shall see) via the arterial blood. However, since the kidneys produce renin and since renal tissue also contains both angiotensinogen and converting enzyme, it is probable that the reactions generating angiotensin I and, in turn, angiotensin II, occur to some extent within the kidneys. Accordingly, the kidneys can probably be influenced not only by blood-borne angiotensin II but also by angiotensin II produced intrarenally.

As we shall see in subsequent chapters, angiotensin II exerts an immense number of effects on diverse tissues, but the end results of most of them are to increase arterial blood pressure. A crucial generalization to be gained from the biochemistry of this system is that because angiotensinogen and converting enzyme are usually present in relatively unchanging concentration, the primary determinant of the rate of angiotensin II formation is the plasma concentration of renin, which is physiologically regulated via the control of renin secretion (to be described in Chapter 5).

The renin-angiotensin system is among the most intensively studied fields in the biomedical sciences, and its biochemistry is proving to be far more complex than the simple description shown in Figure 1-1. Just a few of the important additional findings are as follows: (1) An inactive form of renin with a larger molecular weight is present in plasma, and probably represents the prohormone form of renin (prorenin) initially synthesized by the kidneys; (2) renin or renin-like proteins are produced in sites other than the kidneys (e.g., in the uterus and brain) and may catalyze local generation of angiotensin in these sites; (3) clinically important situations exist in which changes in the concentrations of angiotensinogen or converting enzyme occur and may significantly influence the generation of angiotensin at any given concentration of renin (e.g., oral contraceptives may cause a large increase in plasma angiotensinogen); and (4) angiotensin II can be split to yield the heptapeptide known as angiotensin III, which is also quite active biologically although its relative contribution compared to that of angiotensin II is probably small in most tissues (the enzyme that mediates the generation of angiotensin III seems to be located mainly in the target tissues for this peptide).

Other Vasoactive Substances   In addition to their regulation of salt balance and secretion of renin, the kidneys may exert a third important influence over arterial blood pressure. It is very likely that they either secrete into the blood or remove from it vasoactive substances other than renin. Certainly the kidneys are capable of synthesizing a number of prostaglandins (see below), both vasodilator and vasoconstrictor in action, and the possibility that one or more of these prostaglandins may reach the systemic arterial blood in amounts adequate to dilate or constrict arterioles is the subject of considerable investigation. Secreted lipids other than prostaglandins have also been implicated in the renal regulation of arterial blood pressure.

Regulation of Erythrocyte Production

The kidneys secrete another hormone, erythropoietin, which is involved in the control of erythrocyte production by the bone marrow. Just which renal cells secrete erythropoietin is not yet clear, but the stimulus for its secretion is a decrease in oxygen delivery to the kidneys (as, for example, in anemia, hypoxia, or inadequate renal blood flow). Erythropoietin stimulates the bone marrow to increase its production of erythrocytes. Erythropoietin will not be described further in this book; suffice it to say that renal disease may result in diminished erythropoietin secretion, and the ensuing decrease in bone marrow activity is one important causal factor in the anemia of chronic renal disease.

Regulation of Vitamin D Activity

The kidneys produce the active form of vitamin D (1,25-dihydroxyvitamin D_3). This makes still another hormone secreted by the kidneys; its synthesis and role in calcium metabolism will be described in Chap. 10.

Gluconeogenesis

During prolonged fasting, the kidneys synthesize glucose from amino acids and other precursors and release it into the blood. Thus, like the liver, they are gluconeogenic organs.

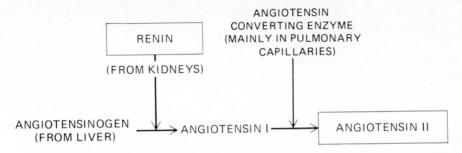

Figure 1-1 Basic biochemistry of renin-angiotensin system.

STRUCTURE OF THE KIDNEYS AND URINARY SYSTEM

The kidneys are paired organs which lie outside the peritoneal cavity in the posterior abdominal wall, one on each side of the vertebral column. The medial border of the kidney is indented by a deep fissure (called the *hilum*) through which pass the renal vessels and nerves and in which lies the funnel-shaped continuation of the upper end of the ureter, the *renal pelvis* (Fig. 1-2). The outer convex border of the renal pelvis is divided into major *calyxes,* each of which subdivides into several minor calyxes. Each of the latter is cupped around the projecting apex of a cone-shaped mass of tissue *(a renal pyramid).*

When the kidney is bisected from top to bottom it can be seen to be divided into two major regions: an inner *renal medulla* and an outer *renal cortex.* The medulla is made up of a number of renal pyramids, the apexes of which, as stated above, project into the minor calyxes. Each pyramid of the medulla, topped by a region of renal cortex, forms a single lobe.

Upon closer gross examination, additional features can be discerned: (1) The cortex has a highly granular appearance missing from the medulla; (2) each medullary pyramid is divisible into an *outer zone* (adjacent to the cortex) and an *inner zone,* including the apical tip (called the *papilla*). All these distinctions reflect the arrangement of the various components of the microscopic subunits of the kidneys, to which we now turn.

The Nephron

In humans, each kidney is composed of approximately 1 million tiny units, *nephrons,* one of which is shown diagrammatically in Fig. 1-3. Each nephron consists of a filtering component, called the *glomerulus*, and a *tubule* extending out from the glomerulus. Let us begin with the glomerulus, which is responsible for the initial step in urine formation, the separation of a protein-free filtrate from plasma.

The Glomerulus The glomerulus consists of a compact tuft of interconnected capillary loops (the *glomerular capillaries*) and a balloonlike hollow capsule (*Bowman's capsule*) into which the capillary tuft protrudes

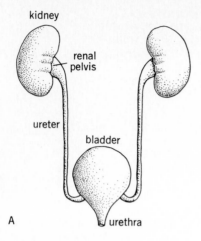

A

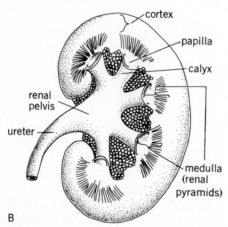

B

Figure 1-2 *a.* The urinary system. The urine, formed by the kidney, collects in the renal pelvis and then flows through the ureter into the bladder, from which it is eliminated via the urethra. *b.* Section of a human kidney. Half the kidney has been sliced away. Note that the structure shows regional differences. The outer portion (cortex), which has a granular appearance, contains all the glomeruli. The collecting ducts form a large portion of the inner kidney (medulla), giving it a striped, pyramidlike appearance, and drain into the renal pelvis. The papilla is the inner portion of the medulla. (*From A. J. Vander et al., Human Physiology,* © *1970 by McGraw-Hill, Inc. Used with permission of McGraw-Hill Book Company.*)

(Fig. 1-4).[1] One way of visualizing the relationship between the glomerular capillaries and Bowman's capsule is to imagine a loosely clenched fist (the capillaries) punched into a balloon (Bowman's capsule). The part of Bowman's capsule in contact with the glomerular capillaries becomes pushed inward but does not make contact with the opposite side of the capsule; accordingly, a space (*Bowman's space*) still exists within the capsule, and it is into this space that fluid filters from the glomerular capillaries across the combined capillary–Bowman's capsule membranes.

This filtration barrier consists of three layers: capillary endothelium, basement membrane, and the single-celled layer of capsular epithelial cells

---

[1] There is no complete agreement as to whether the glomerulus should refer only to the capillary tuft or to the tuft plus Bowman's capsule; the latter is presently the more common usage.

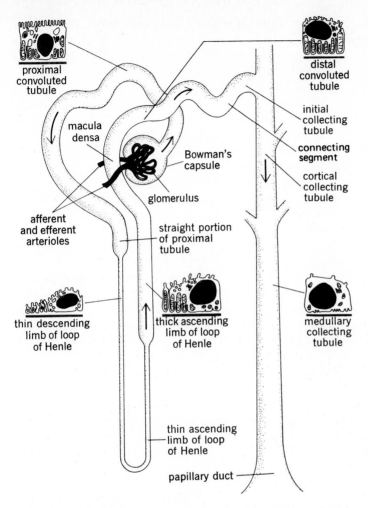

proximal
convoluted
tubule

distal
convoluted
tubule

macula
densa

initial
collecting
tubule

connecting
segment

Bowman's
capsule

cortical
collecting
tubule

glomerulus

afferent
and efferent
arterioles

straight portion
of proximal
tubule

thin descending
limb of loop
of Henle

thick ascending
limb of loop
of Henle

medullary
collecting
tubule

thin ascending
limb of loop
of Henle

papillary duct

Figure 1-3 Relationships of component parts of a long-looped nephron, which has been "uncoiled" for clarity; relative lengths of the different segments are not accurate. [*Drawings of fine structure adapted from J. Rhodin, Int. Rev. Cytol., 7:485(1958).*] This nephron is either a midcortical or juxtamedullary nephron (see Fig. 1-5).

(Fig. 1-4). The first layer, the endothelial cells of the capillaries, is perforated by many large fenestrae. The basement membrane is a relatively homogenous acellular meshwork of glycoproteins and mucopolysaccharides. The epithelial cells resting on the basement membrane are quite different from the relatively simple, flattened cells lining the rest of Bowman's capsule (the part of the "balloon" not in contact with the "fist") and are called *podocytes;* they have an unusual octopuslike structure in that they possess a large number of extensions, or *foot processes,* which are embedded in the basement membrane, foot processes from adjacent podocytes manifesting a great degree of interdigitation. *Slits* exist between adjacent foot processes and constitute the path through which the filtrate, once through the endothelial cells and basement membrane, travels to enter Bowman's space. However, for two reasons, these slits do not offer completely open passageways: (1) The foot processes are coated by a thick layer of extracellular material (glycosialoproteins), which partially occludes the slits; (2) extremely thin diaphragms bridge the slits at the surface of the basement membrane.

The functional significance of this anatomical arrangement is that blood in the glomerular capillaries is separated from Bowman's space by only a thin set of membranes, which permits the filtration of fluid from the capillaries into the space. Bowman's capsule connects at the side opposite the glomerular tuft with the first portion of the tubule, into which this filtered fluid then flows.

Our discussion of the glomerulus has focused on the two types of cells —capillary endothelium and podocytes—in the filtration barrier. However, there is a third cell type—*mesangial cells*—found in the central part of the glomerular tuft between and within capillary loops. Certain of the glomerular mesangial cells act as phagocytes, whereas others contain large numbers of myofilaments and are able to contract in response to a variety of stimuli. The role such contraction plays in influencing filtration through the glomeruli will be discussed in Chap. 5.

The Tubule   Throughout its course, the tubule is composed of a single layer of epithelial cells resting on a basement membrane. The structure and function of these epithelial cells vary considerably from segment to segment of the tubule, but one common feature is the presence of tight junctions between adjacent cells.

Physiologists and anatomists have traditionally grouped two or more continuous tubular segments for purposes of reference, but unfortunately the terminologies used in these disciplines have not been identical. Table 1-2 lists the various nephron segments (they are illustrated in Fig. 1-5) and the combination terms used by most physiologists.

The segment of the tubule that drains Bowman's capsule is the *proximal tubule* (Fig. 1-3), which initially forms several coils (the *convoluted portion,* or *pars convoluta,* of the proximal tubule) followed by a straight segment (*pars recta*), which descends toward the medulla. (Although it is traditional to divide the proximal tubule into two segments—the pars convoluta and the pars recta—there are actually three histologically distinguishable segments: S_1, which includes the first part of the pars convoluta; S_2, which includes the rest of the pars convoluta and the first portion of the pars recta; and S_3, the rest of the pars recta.)

The next segment, into which the pars recta drains, is the *descending thin limb of the loop of Henle.* (Anatomists traditionally consider the

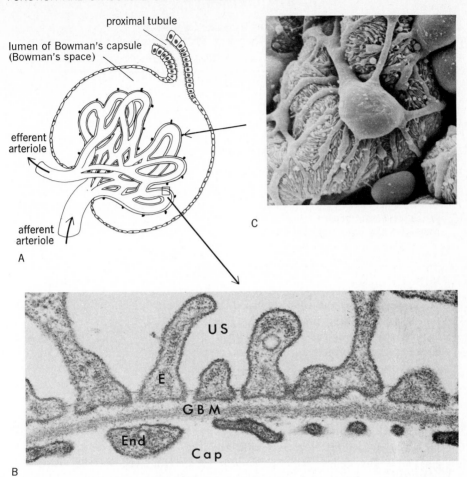

Figure 1-4 *a.* Anatomy of the glomerulus. *b.* Cross section of glomerular membranes US = "Urinary" (Bowman's) space, E = epithelial foot processes, GBM = glomerular basement membranes, End = capillary endothelium, Cap = lumen of capillary. Note the basement membrane is itself not homogenous but has a denser core. [*Courtesy H. G. Rennke; orginally published in Fed. proc.,* **36**:*2619(1977); reprinted with permission*]. *c.* Scanning electron micrograph of podocytes covering glomerular capillary loops; the view is from inside Bowman's space. The large mass is a cell body. Note the remarkable interdigitation of the foot processes from adjacent podocytes and the slits between them. (*Courtesy of Dr. Craig Tisher.*)

pars recta as the first portion of the loop of Henle, whereas physiologists consider it the last portion of the proximal tubule, as shown in Table 1-2.)

At the hairpin turn, the *ascending limb of the loop of Henle* begins, and a transition occurs in the epithelium. In long loops (see below), the first portion of the ascending limb remains *thin* (but different from the

Table 1-2 Terms Used to Denote Tubular Segments

Sequence of Distinct Segments	Combination Terms
Proximal convoluted tubule (pars convoluta)	Proximal tubule
Proximal straight tubule (pars recta)	
Descending thin limb of loop of Henle	
Ascending thin limb of loop of Henle	
Medullary thick ascending limb of loop of Henle	Loop of Henle
Cortical thick ascending limb of loop of Henle	
Macula densa	
Distal convoluted tubule	Distal tubule
Connecting tubule	
Initial collecting tubule	
Cortical collecting tubule	
Outer medullary collecting tubule	Collecting duct
Inner medullary collecting tubule	
Papillary collecting duct	

descending limb), and then the upper portion becomes *thick;* in short loops, the entire ascending limb is thick (Fig. 1-5).

At the end of the ascending limb of Henle's loop, the tubule passes between the arterioles supplying its glomerulus of origin (Fig. 1-3); this very short segment is known as the *macula densa*. Beyond the macula densa is the *distal tubule*, traditionally defined by micropuncturists as the segment between the macula densa and the first junction of two tubules. However, the distal tubule is not a homogenous unit, either structurally or functionally. It is really a zone of transition between the thick ascending loop of Henle and the collecting system. The early portion is the coiled *distal convoluted tubule*, followed by the *connecting segment* (or *connecting tubule)*, and then the *initial collecting tubule* (not all nephrons have both of these last two subsegments). The connecting tubule and initial collecting tubule are often called the *late distal tubule*.

From the glomerulus to the ends of the distal convoluted tubules, each of the 1 million tubules in each kidney is completely separate from the others. Depending upon the location in the kidney, connecting segments and/or initial collecting tubules join end to end or side to side to form *cortical collecting tubules*. These run downward to enter the medulla and become *medullary collecting tubules*, the last portion of which are called *papillary collecting ducts*, which empty into a calyx of the renal pelvis. The calyx is continuous with the *ureter*, which empties into the *urinary bladder*, where urine is temporarily stored and from which it is intermittently eliminated. The urine is not altered after it enters a calyx. From this point on, the remainder of the urinary system simply serves as plumbing.

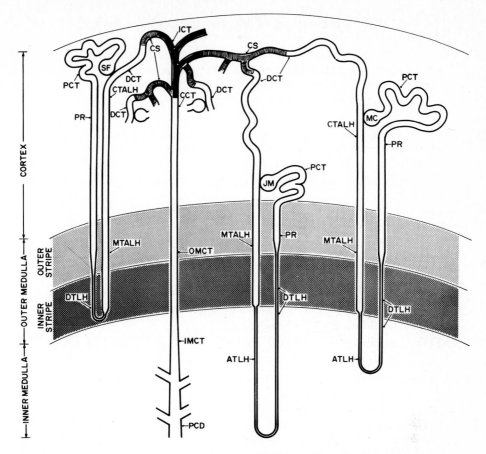

Figure 1-5 Three populations of nephrons, based on location of their glomeruli, are schematically depicted: superficial (SF), midcortical (MC), and juxtamedullary(JM). The major nephron segments are labeled as follows: PCT, proximal convoluted tubule; PR, pars recta; DTLH, descending thin limb of Henle; ATLH, ascending thin limb of Henle; MTALH, medullary thick ascending limb of Henle; CTALH, cortical thick ascending limb of Henle; DCT, distal convoluted tubule; CS, connecting segment; ICT, initial collecting tubule; CCT, cortical collecting tubule; OMCT, outer medullary collecting tubule; IMCT, inner medullary collecting tubule; PCD, papillary collecting duct. [From H. R. Jacobson, *Am. J. Physiol.*, **241**: F203(1981).]

Blood Supply to the Nephrons

In the earlier section on the glomerulus, we described the glomerular capillaries but made no mention of their origin. Blood enters each kidney via a renal artery, which then divides into progressively smaller branches — interlobar, arcuate, and finally interlobular arteries. Each of the interlobular arteries gives off at right angles to itself, as it courses toward the kidney surface, a parallel series of *afferent arterioles* (Figs. 1-3 and 1-5), each of which leads to a glomerulus. (Thus, the afferent arteriole is the "arm" to which the "fist" is attached.)

Normally, only about 20 percent of the plasma (and none of the erythrocytes) entering the glomerular capillaries is filtered into Bowman's capsule; where does the remaining blood go next? In almost all other organs, capillaries recombine to form the beginnings of the venous system. The glomerular capillaries instead recombine to form another set of arterioles called the *efferent arterioles*. Thus, blood leaves each glomerulus through a single efferent arteriole, which soon subdivides into a second set of capillaries (Fig. 1-6). These *peritubular capillaries* are profusely distributed to, and intimately associated with, all the portions of the tubule, an arrangement which permits movement of solutes and water between the tubular lumen and capillaries. They rejoin to form the venous channels by which blood ultimately leaves the kidney.

Interestingly, in general, the efferent vessel (and peritubular capillaries arising from it) from a given glomerulus are dissociated from the tubule originating from that glomerulus, i.e., the efferent arteriole supplies a different tubule. Moreover, the various segments of any single tubule are supplied with blood coming from multiple efferent arterioles.

Regional Differences in Structure

There are important regional differences in the locations of the various tubular and vascular components. The cortex contains all the glomeruli (this accounts for its granular appearance), proximal and distal tubules, cortical collecting tubules, and cortical portions of the loops of Henle.

Nephrons are categorized according to the locations of their glomeruli in the cortex (Fig. 1-5): (1) *superficial cortical nephrons* have glomeruli located within 1 mm of the capsular surface of the kidneys; (2) *midcortical nephrons* have glomeruli located, as their name states, in the midcortex, deep to the superficial cortical nephrons but above the next category; (3) *juxtamedullary nephrons* (sometimes called inner cortical nephrons) have their glomeruli located just above the corticomedullary junction. One major distinction between these three categories is the length of the loop of Henle. All superficial cortical nephrons have short loops of Henle, which make their turn superficial to the junction of outer and inner medulla. All juxtamedullary nephrons have long loops, which extend into the inner medulla, often to the tip of a papilla. Midcortical nephrons may be either short-looped or long-looped. The additional length of the loop of Henle in long-looped nephrons is due entirely to the length of the thin segments. Finally, the beginning of the thick ascending limb in the longest loops marks the border between outer and inner medulla.

The three nephron populations differ from each other structurally in ways other than the lengths of their loops of Henle; moreover, the midcortical nephrons themselves are not homogenous but manifest gradations of structural characteristics as one moves inward. It seems certain that all this structural heterogeneity is reflected in functional heterogeneity.

The vascular structures supplying the medulla also differ (Fig. 1-6). In the inner portions of the cortex, many glomeruli have long efferent arterioles, which extend to the outer medulla where they divide many times to form *vascular bundles*. The margins of these bundles give rise to a capillary network which surrounds loops of Henle and collecting ducts in the outer medulla. From the cores of the bundles, straight vessels (*descending vasa recta*) extend to the inner medulla, where they break up into a capillary plexus. These inner medullary capillaries re-form into veins (*ascending vasa recta*) which run in close association with the descending vasa recta within the vascular bundles. This relationship, as we shall see, has considerable significance for the formation of a concentrated urine.

Note also (Fig. 1-6) that some of the blood vessels originating in juxtamedullary nephrons do not supply cortical structures. As will be discussed later, this is important for explaining why some chemical methods used for measuring renal blood flow provide underestimates.

One other regional difference concerns so-called *interstitial cells*, which become more numerous and larger as one descends from cortex to papilla. These cells, which are located between adjacent tubules and capillaries, are thought to be one site for the synthesis of prostaglandins.

The Juxtaglomerular Apparatus

Reference was made earlier to the macula densa, that portion of the tubule which marks the boundary between the ascending loop of Henle and the distal convoluted tubule. In all nephrons, this segment courses between the afferent and efferent arterioles at the hilus of the glomerulus of the macula densa's own nephron. This entire area is known as the *juxtaglomerular (JG) apparatus* (Fig. 1-7). (Don't confuse the term "juxtaglomerular apparatus" with "juxtamedullary nephron.") Each JG apparatus is composed of three cell types: (1) *granular cells*, which appear to be differentiated smooth muscle cells in the walls of the arterioles (particularly in the afferent arterioles); (2) extraglomerular mesangial cells; and (3) the macula densa cells. The granular cells (so-called because they contain secretory vesicles) are the cells that secrete the hormone renin, mentioned earlier in this chapter. The extraglomerular mesangial cells are morphologically similar to and continuous with the intraglomerular mesangial cells described earlier. The function of these extraglomerular mesangial cells is unknown, but there is some evidence that they communicate with granular cells via gap junctions and that they may be transformed into granular cells with appropriate physiological stimuli (indeed, granular cells are found scattered within the mesangium). The macula densa is in contact with the vascular component of the juxtaglomerular apparatus, and the macula densa cells (and/or the early distal tubular cells beyond the macula densa) probably contribute

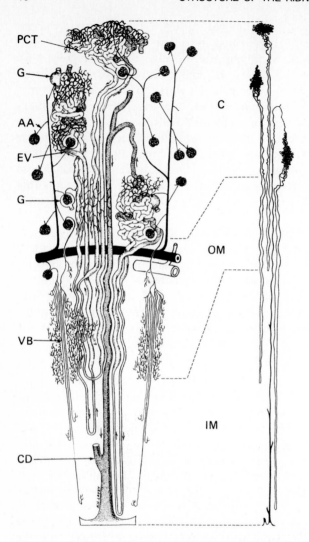

Figure 1-6 Diagram of renal vascular and tubular organization. Only three nephrons (one from each general population) are shown, vascular structures are extensively simplified, and vertical scale is compressed. The same nephrons are shown undistorted to the right. Major zones are: cortex (C), outer medulla (OM), and inner medulla (IM). Afferent arterioles (AA), glomeruli (G), and efferent vessels (EV) are shown together with part of the peritubular capillary network. The proximal convoluted tubules (PCT) and distal convoluted tubules (dark hatching) are generally dissociated from the efferent network arising from their parent glomeruli. Some midcortical efferents directly perfuse Henle loops and collecting ducts in cortical medullary rays. In outer medulla, descending thin limbs of short loops are close to vascular bundles (VB), while thin limbs of long loops are found with thick ascending limbs and collecting ducts (CD) in the interbundle region. Note the relationships of the capillary plexuses (CP) to the vascular bundles. [*Courtesy of Reiner Beeuwkes III; Adapted from Am. J. Physiol.*, **229**:*695 (1975)*.]

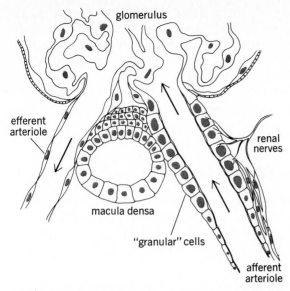

glomerulus

efferent
arteriole

renal
nerves

macula densa

"granular" cells

afferent
arteriole

Figure 1-7 Diagram of glomerulus showing the juxtaglomerular apparatus. The granular cells secrete renin and are also thought to function as baroreceptors; mesangial cells are not shown. [*Redrawn from J. O. Davis, Am. J. Med.,* **55**:*333(1973)*.]

both to the control of renin secretion and to the control of glomerular filtration rate (as will be described in Chap. 5).

Finally, there is a rich supply of sympathetic neurons to the various structures of the juxtaglomerular apparatus.

INTRARENAL CHEMICAL MESSENGERS

As we shall see in subsequent chapters, the kidneys are the target organs for multiple neural and hormonal inputs. In addition, in response to appropriate stimuli, the kidneys themselves synthesize a variety of substances which function as intrarenal chemical messengers. The biochemistry of several of these will be described briefly here, and their postulated functions will be dealt with in subsequent chapters.

As pointed out earlier, intrarenally generated angiotensin II is one such substance. So are the prostaglandins. The kidneys are capable of producing a large number of prostaglandins (including PGE_2, $PGF_2\alpha$, PGD_2, thromboxane A_2, and prostacyclin). There are some differences in the types of prostaglandins produced by cells of cortical and medullary structures,[2] but probably no sharp demarcation.

[2] In the cortex, the sites of production are the endothelial cells lining arteries and arterioles, the glomeruli, and the cortical collecting ducts. In the medulla, interstitial cells and collecting ducts are the major sites.

A third group of intrarenally generated chemical messengers is the *kinins*, the collective name given to *lysyl bradykinin* and *bradykinin*. The kinins are peptides released from plasma protein precursors by several plasma and tissue enzymes called *kallikreins*. The specific kallikrein produced and secreted by the kidneys (by cells of the distal tubule) splits lysyl bradykinin from plasma kininogen, and lysyl bradykinin is cleaved again within the kidneys to yield bradykinin (note the analogies between the kallikrein-kinin and renin-angiotensin systems).

Perhaps the most fascinating (and confusing) features of the renin-angiotensin system, the renal prostaglandins, and the renal kallikrein-kinin system is the host of interactions being discovered among these three groups of chemical messengers. Only those interactions considered best established and important will be described in subsequent chapters, but the interested reader may obtain more information by consulting the Suggested Readings.

Finally, these three complex groups by no means exhaust the list of likely intrarenal chemical messengers, and several others will be mentioned later.

METHODS IN RENAL PHYSIOLOGY

Because of its limited scope and objectives, this book will deal very little with the methods used to study renal physiology. Only the method known as "clearance" is described to any extent (in Chap. 3) because of its widespread clinical use. Another technique which has been a mainstay of renal physiologists is *micropuncture*, the insertion of a micropipette into a nephron segment to withdraw fluid for analysis. This technique was originally established for use in amphibians, whose nephrons are relatively large and can be seen easily since they are not packed together into an enclosed organ. Micropuncture has since been used to withdraw fluid from various nephron segments of mammalian kidneys, as well as to measure pressures, perfuse tubules, and perform other manipulations on single nephrons in situ. A third technique is that of perfusing isolated separated segments of a single nephron in vitro, and this is making possible many studies that could not be done with older techniques. For example, micropuncture is generally applicable only to the most superficial nephrons since these can be visualized by looking down upon the surface of the kidney. This had been a major impediment to studying medullary structures and functional heterogeneity of nephrons.

In addition to clearance, micropuncture, and the isolated, perfused tubule, a plethora of other useful techniques has been developed, and all of them, like the "big three," have particular advantages and disadvantages. The interested reader should consult the list of Suggested Readings at the back of the book.

Study questions: 1 and 2

CHAPTER 2

BASIC RENAL PROCESSES

OBJECTIVES

The student knows the basic principles of renal physiology.

1 Lists and defines the three basic renal processes: glomerular filtration, tubular reabsorption, tubular secretion
2 Describes the routes for blood and fluid movements within the kidneys
3 Describes the chemical characteristics of the glomerular filtrate
4 States the sites in the glomerulus for restriction of macromolecules; defines steric hindrance and electrical hindrance and relates them to protein filtration; describes glomerular "sieving"
5 States the formula for the determinants of glomerular net filtration pressure and the normal values for each determinant; states how several of these values change along the length of the glomerular capillaries
6 Defines filtration pressure equilibrium
7 States the factors determining glomerular filtration rate; defines hydraulic permeability and filtration coefficient (K_f)
8 States how mesangial cells alter K_f
9 Describes how arterial pressure, afferent-arteriolar resistance, and efferent-arteriolar resistance determine glomerular-capillary pressure
10 States the effect of obstruction on P_{BC}
11 Describes the determinants of π_{GC} and how the rate of plasma flow influences this variable
12 Predicts the direction of change of GFR under a variety of situations, including hypotension, reduced plasma protein concentration, and ureteral occlusion

13   Defines and states the major characteristics of simple facilitated diffusion, secondary active transport, primary active transport, and endocytosis

14   States how the mechanisms of Objective 13 can be combined to achieve net transepithelial movement (i.e., net reabsorption or secretion)

15   Defines the concept of T_m (either reabsorptive or secretory); given appropriate data, calculates T_m; defines threshold; defines splay and describes the mechanism for it; states the significance of a T_m being much higher than the usual filtered mass of the substance

16   Defines "pump-leak" system and states its consequences

17   Contrasts "tight" and "leaky" epithelia

Urine formation begins with the filtration of essentially protein-free plasma through the glomerular capillaries into Bowman's capsule. The final urine that enters the renal pelvis is quite different from the *glomerular filtrate* because, as the filtered fluid flows from Bowman's capsule through the various portions of the tubule, its composition is altered. This change occurs by two general processes: tubular reabsorption and tubular secretion. The tubule is at all points intimately associated with the peritubular capillaries, a relationship that permits transfer of materials between the peritubular-capillary plasma and the lumen of the tubule. When the direction of transfer is from tubular lumen to peritubular-capillary plasma, the process is called *tubular reabsorption.* Movement in the opposite direction, i.e., from peritubular-capillary plasma to tubular lumen, is called *tubular secretion.* This last term must not be confused with *excretion.* To say that a substance has been excreted is to say that it appears in the final urine. These relationships are illustrated in Fig. 2-1.

The most common relationships between these basic renal processes —glomerular filtration, tubular reabsorption, and tubular secretion—are shown in Fig. 2-2. Plasma, containing substances X, Y, and Z, enters the glomerular capillaries. A certain quantity of protein-free plasma containing these substances is filtered into Bowman's capsule, enters the proximal tubule, and begins its flow through the rest of the tubule. The remainder of the plasma, also containing X, Y, and Z, leaves the glomerular capillaries via an efferent arteriole and enters the peritubular capillaries. The cells composing the tubular epithelium can transport X (not Y or Z) from the peritubular plasma into the tubular lumen but not in the opposite direction. By this combination of filtration and tubular secretion, all the plasma that originally entered the renal artery is cleared of substance X, which leaves the body via the urine, thus reducing the amount of X remaining in the body. If the tubule were incapable of reabsorption, the Y and Z originally filtered at the glomerulus would also leave the body via the urine, but the tubule can, in fact, reabsorb Y and Z. The amount of this reabsorption of Y is small, so most of the filtered material does escape from the body. But for Z the reabsorptive mechanism is so powerful that virtually all

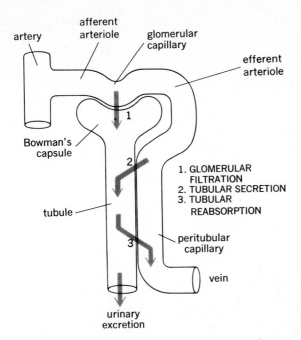

Figure 2-1 The three basic components of renal function. *(From A. J. Vander et al., Human Physiology, © 1970 by McGraw-Hill, Inc. Used with permission of McGraw-Hill Book Company.)*

the filtered material is reabsorbed back into the plasma, which then flows through the renal vein back into the vena cava. Therefore, no Z is lost from the body. Hence, the processes of filtration and reabsorption have canceled each other, and the net result is as though Z had never entered the kidney at all.

The kidney works only on plasma; the erythrocytes supply oxygen to the kidney but serve no other function in urine formation. Each substance in plasma is handled in a characteristic manner by the nephron, i.e., by a particular combination of filtration, reabsorption, and secretion. (Tubular synthesis with subsequent release of the synthesized products into either the blood or the tubular lumen might well be listed as a fourth basic renal process; for example, we shall see that the tubular cells synthesize ammonia.) The critical point is that *the rates at which the relevant basic processes proceed for many of these substances are subject to physiological control.* What is the effect, for example, if the filtered mass of Y is increased or its reabsorption rate decreased? Either change causes more Y to be lost from the body via the urine. By triggering changes in the rates of filtration, reabsorption, or secretion whenever the plasma concentration of a substance goes above or below normal, homeostatic mechanisms regulate the plasma concentration of the substance.

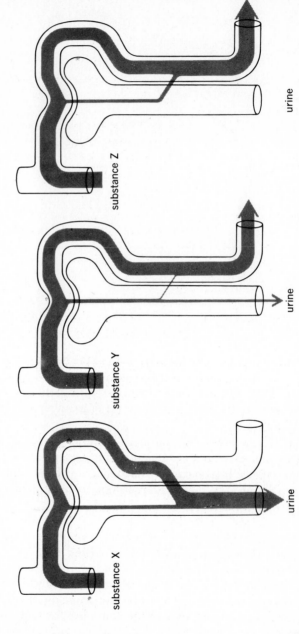

Figure 2-2 Renal manipulation of three substances, X, Y, and Z. X is filtered and secreted but not reabsorbed. Y is filtered, and a fraction is then reabsorbed. Z is filtered but is completely reabsorbed. (*From A. J. Vander et al., Human Physiology,* © *1970 by McGraw-Hill, Inc. Used with permission of McGraw-Hill Book Company.*)

In summary, one can study the normal renal handling of any given substance by asking a series of questions:

1 To what degree is the substance filterable at the glomerulus?

2 Is it reabsorbed?

3 Is it secreted?

4 What are the mechanisms by which reabsorption or secretion is achieved?

5 What factors homeostatically regulate the quantities filtered, reabsorbed, or secreted, i.e., what are the pathways by which renal excretion of the substance is altered so as to maintain stable body balance?

6 What factors other than renal disease can perturb body balance of the substance by causing the kidneys to filter, reabsorb, or secrete too much or too little of the substance?

For clinicians, of course, a seventh question must be asked: How do the various types of renal disease influence the handling of the substance and its total body balance?

GLOMERULAR FILTRATION

In a normal 70-kg person, the average volume of fluid filtered from the plasma into Bowman's capsule is 180 L/day (approximately 45 gal)! The implications of this remarkable fact are extremely important. When we recall that the average total volume of plasma in humans is approximately 3 L, it follows that the entire plasma volume is filtered by the kidneys some 60 times a day. It is, in part, this ability to process such huge volumes of plasma that enables the kidneys to excrete large quantities of waste products and to regulate the constituents of the internal environment so precisely. The second implication concerns the magnitude of the reabsorption process. The average person excretes between 1 and 2 L of urine per day. Since 180 L of fluid are filtered, approximately 99 percent of the filtered water must have been reabsorbed into the peritubular capillaries, the remaining 1 percent escaping from the body as urinary water.

Composition of the Filtrate

The glomerular capillaries are freely permeable to water and to *crystalloids,* i.e., solutes of small molecular dimensions. They are relatively impermeable to large molecules or *colloids,* the most important of which are the plasma proteins. Therefore, the fluid within Bowman's capsule is essentially protein-free and contains most crystalloids in virtually the same concentrations as in the plasma.[1] These facts were established by micropuncture. Any crystalloid that is partially bound to protein has a lower concentration in Bowman's capsule than in the plasma because the protein-bound moiety will not filter out of the capillary. For such a substance, the concentration in Bowman's capsule will equal the plasma concentration not bound to protein.

The phrase "essentially protein-free" has been used several times in referring to the glomerular filtrate. The fact is that the glomerular filtrate is not completely protein-free but does contain extremely small quantities of protein (almost entirely albumin), on the order of 50 mg/L or less. (This is less than 0.1 percent of the concentration of protein in plasma.) This protein crosses the glomerular membranes to reach Bowman's space by carriage along with the other components of the filtrate and by simple diffusion. In various disease states, the glomerular membranes may be altered so as to permit marked increases in the passage of protein into Bowman's space. Moreover, even in the absence of glomerular alteration, when certain small proteins not normally present in the plasma appear there because of disease (for example, hemoglobin released from damaged erythrocytes, and myoglobin released from damaged muscles), considerable filtration of them may occur.

This emphasizes that the glomerular membranes behave as all-or-none filters only with regard to crystalloids and large proteins. There is no hindrance to the movement of molecules with molecular weights less than 7000; beyond this, "sieving" begins and progressively increases, becoming essentially total for plasma albumin.

Nature of the Glomerular Barrier to Macromolecules

The route that filtered substances take through the glomerular membranes — fenestra in the endothelial layer, basement membrane, slit diaphragms, and slits — is completely extracellular. Most of the restriction to macromolecules takes place in the basement membrane, in the hydrated spaces between the elongated, intertwining glycoprotein chains constituting this gel-like layer. However, restriction by this primary filter is not absolute for most macromolecules, and some that do traverse the entire thickness of the basement membrane encounter further restriction both by the slit diaphragms and the coats of the podocytes, which occupy much of the slits. (This is a good time to reread the glomerular anatomy section of Chap. 1.) The reader might well wonder what happens to macromolecules that get hung up at

---

[1] Actually, the concentrations of charged crystalloids in Bowman's capsule are not exactly the same as in plasma water, because the presence of the plasma proteins causes a Donnan equilibrium to exist between these fluids, but this effect is small and may be ignored.

these sites; they are probably taken into the foot processes by endocytosis and broken down.

The discussion thus far has dealt only with steric hindrance, i.e., impairment of macromolecular movement solely because of size. However, electric charge is also a critical variable in determining penetration by proteins and other macromolecules. The molecules that constitute the extracellular matrix of the glomerular barrier (the cell coats of the endothelium, the basement membrane, and the cell coats of the podocytes) are almost all polyanions. Accordingly, for any given size, negatively charged macromolecules are restricted more than neutral molecules are from entering and moving through the wall, because the fixed polyanions repel the negatively charged molecules. (It is useful to imagine simply that the route followed constitutes "pores" lined with negative charges.) Since almost all proteins bear net negative charges, this electrical hindrance plays an important restrictive role, enhancing that of purely steric hindrance. It is very likely that many of the diseases that cause glomeruli to be "leaky" to protein eliminate many of the negative charges in the wall. It must be emphasized that these negative charges act as a hindrance only to macromolecules, not to the plasma crystalloids, which are too small to be significantly influenced by any charges "lining the pores."

Forces Involved in Filtration: Net Filtration Pressure

The *net filtration pressure* (NFP) for any capillary is the algebraic sum of the opposing hydraulic and colloid osmotic (oncotic) pressures acting across the capillary. This also applies to the glomerular capillaries:

$$NFP = \underbrace{(P_{GC} + \pi_{BC})}_{\text{forces inducing filtration}} - \underbrace{(P_{BC} + \pi_{GC})}_{\text{forces opposing filtration}}$$

where P_{GC} = glomerular-capillary hydraulic pressure

π_{BC} = oncotic pressure of fluid in Bowman's capsule

P_{BC} = hydraulic pressure in Bowman's capsule

π_{GC} = oncotic pressure in glomerular-capillary plasma

Because there is virtually no protein in Bowman's capsule, π_{BC} may be taken as zero so that the equation becomes (Fig. 2-3):

$$NFP = P_{GC} - P_{BC} - \pi_{GC}$$

The hydraulic pressures in glomerular capillaries and Bowman's capsule have not been directly measured in people. However, several lines of indirect evidence suggest that the human values are probably similar to those for the dog, and the latter are shown in Table 2-1 and Fig. 2-4a, along with

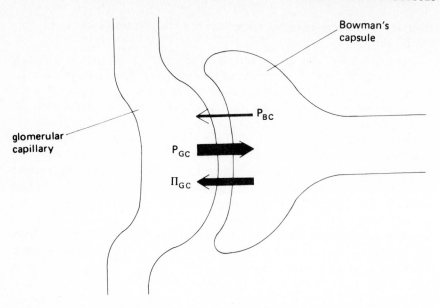

Figure 2-3 Net filtration pressure at the glomerulus equals glomerular-capillary hydraulic pressure (P_{GC}) minus Bowman's capsule hydraulic pressure (P_{BC}) minus glomerular-capillary oncotic pressure (π_{GC}).

glomerular capillary oncotic pressure. Note that both the hydraulic and oncotic pressures in the glomerular capillaries change along the length of the capillaries: (1) Capillary hydraulic pressure decreases slightly because of the resistance to flow offered by the capillaries; (2) oncotic pressure increases because, since the filtrate is essentially protein-free, the filtration process removes water but not protein from the plasma, thereby increasing the protein concentration of the unfiltered plasma remaining in the glomerular capillaries. In dogs, approximately 30 percent of the plasma water is normally filtered, but the resulting rise in glomerular-capillary oncotic pressure exceeds 30 percent because, for physicochemical reasons we will not discuss, the relationship between oncotic pressure and plasma protein concentration is not linear.

Fig. 2-4a and Table 2-1 show that, in the dog, net filtration pressure is 24 mmHg at the beginning of the glomerular capillaries and 10 mmHg at the end. As stated above, these values are probably a reasonable approximation of those for normal human beings. However, because this is by no means a certainty, it should at least be noted that in all species of experimental animals directly studied, other than the dog, glomerular-capillary hydraulic pressure normally is lower than the value observed in dogs; therefore, net filtration pressure is also lower and may actually become zero at some point along the glomerular capillary, a phenomenon known as *filtration pressure*

Table 2-1 Forces Involved in Glomerular Filtration in Dogs

		mmHg	
Forces		Afferent end of glomerular capillary	Efferent end of glomerular capillary
1 Favoring filtration: Glomerular-capillary hydraulic pressure, P_{GC}		60	58
2 Oppossing filtration:			
	a Hydraulic pressure in Bowman's capsule, P_{BC}	15	15
	b Oncotic pressure in glomerular capillary, π_{GC}	21 —	33 —
3 Net filtration pressure [(1) − (2)]		24	10

equilibrium (Fig. 2-4*b*). This situation may also occur in human beings when glomerular-capillary pressure is unusually low, as for example following a severe hemorrhage.

Glomerular Filtration Rate (GFR)

The rate of filtration from glomerular capillaries into Bowman's capsule *(glomerular filtration rate, GFR)* depends not only upon the net filtration pressure (NFP) described in the previous section, but upon both the hydraulic (water) permeability of the glomerular membranes and the surface area available for filtration:

GFR = hydraulic permeability × surface area × NFP

The product of hydraulic permeability and surface area is known as the *filtration coefficient (Kf)*. Accordingly:

$GFR = K_f \times NFP$

Let us expand the equation to reemphasize all its components.

$$GFR = \underset{\substack{\text{(hydraulic permeability} \\ \times \text{ surface area)}}}{K_f} \times \underset{(P_{GC} - P_{BC} - \pi_{GC})}{NFP}$$

As stated earlier, the normal GFR per day for a 70-kg person is 180L (125 ml/min). That a net filtration pressure of approximately 10 to 24 mmHg suffices to filter this huge volume of fluid is attributable to the fact that K_f for glomerular capillaries, relative to nonrenal capillaries, is very large, partly because the glomerular capillaries have a large surface area

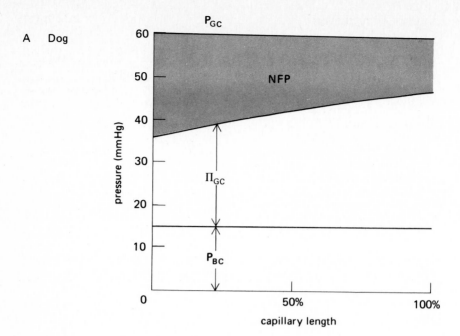

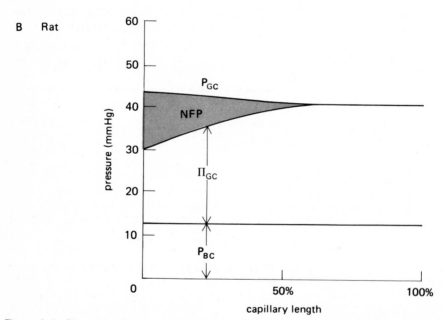

Figure 2-4 Glomerular filtration pressures in dog and rat. Net filtration pressure (NFP) = P_{GC} − (π_{GC} + P_{BC}). Note that in the rat, but not in the dog, NFP becomes zero well before the end of the tubule; i.e., filtration-pressure equilibrium occurs. It is likely that values for human beings are similar to those of the dog, except under certain pathological conditions (see text).

Table 2-2 Summary of Direct GFR Determinants and Factors That Influence Them

Direct determinants of GFR: $GFR = K_f \cdot (P_{GC} - P_{BC} - \pi_{GC})$	Major factors that tend to increase the magnitude of the direct determinant
K_f*	↑ glomerular surface area due to relaxation of glomerular mesangial cells Result: ↑ GFR
P_{GC}*	↑ renal arterial pressure ↓ afferent arteriolar resistance (afferent dilation) ↑ efferent arteriolar resistance (efferent constriction) Result: ↑ GFR
P_{BC}*	↑ intratubular pressure due to obstruction of tubule or extrarenal urinary system Result: ↓ GFR
π_{GC}*	↑ systemic-plasma oncotic pressure (sets π_{GC} at beginnig of glomerular capillaries) ↓ total renal plasma flow (sets rate of rise of π_{GC} along glomerular capillaries) Result: ↓ GFR

*K_f = filtration coefficient; P_{GC} = glomerular-capillary hydraulic pressure; P_{BC} = Bowman's capsule hydraulic pressure; π_{GC} = glomerular-capillary oncotic pressure. A reversal of all arrows in the table will cause a decrease in the magnitudes of K_f, P_{GC}, P_{BC} and π_{GC}.

but, more important, because they have a much greater (10- to 100-fold) hydraulic permeability.

The GFR is not fixed, but may show marked fluctuations in differing physiological states and in disease. If all other factors remain constant, any change in the glomerular hydraulic permeability or surface area, in the hydraulic pressures within the glomerular capillaries or Bowman's capsule, or in the oncotic pressure of glomerular-capillary plasma will alter GFR. The next question becomes: What factors influence these direct determinants of GFR (Table 2-2)?

K_f Changes in K_f can occur in glomerular disease, but only recently has it been recognized that this variable is also subject to physiological control; a variety of chemical mediators cause contraction of glomerular mesangial cells, with a resulting decrease in glomerular surface area and, hence, K_f. This decrease in K_f will tend to lower GFR.[2]

P_{GC}   Glomerular-capillary hydraulic pressure (P_{GC}) is the determinant of GFR under tightest physiological control. P_{GC} reflects the interplay of renal arterial pressure, afferent-arteriolar resistance (R_A), and efferent-arteriolar resistance (R_E). As should be clear from Fig. 2-5, a change in renal arterial pressure will *tend to* cause a change in P_{GC} of the same direction (as will be described in Chap. 5, the use of the phrase "tend to cause" here and elsewhere in this discussion reflects the fact that other simultaneously occurring events my oppose the effect of the specific factor being analyzed). At any given renal arterial pressure, an increase in R_A (afferent-arteriolar constriction) will tend to lower P_{GC} (simply by causing a greater loss of pressure between the renal arteries and glomerular capillaries). Conversely, a decrease in R_A (afferent-arteriolar dilation) will tend to raise P_{GC}. More difficult to visualize is the fact that changes in R_E also tend to cause changes in P_{GC}, changes opposite to those caused by changes in R_A; i.e., an increase in R_E (efferent-arteriolar constriction) tends to elevate P_{GC}. This happens because the efferent arteriole lies beyond the glomerulus, so that efferent-arteriolar constriction tends to "dam back" the blood in the glomerular capillaries, raising P_{GC}. Similarly, a decrease in R_E (efferent-arteriolar dilation) tends to lower P_{GC}.

P_{BC}   The major cause of increased hydraulic pressure in Bowman's capsule is obstruction anywhere along the tubule or in the external portions of the urinary system (ureter, etc.); the effect of such an occlusion is to increase the tubular pressure everywhere proximal to the occlusion, all the way back to Bowman's capsule. The result is to decrease GFR.

π_{GC}   Oncotic pressure in the plasma at the very beginning of the glomerular capillaries is, of course, simply the oncotic pressure of systemic arterial plasma. Accordingly, a decrease in systemic-plasma protein concentration, as occurs for example in liver disease, will lower plasma oncotic pressure and tend to increase GFR.

But now recall (Fig. 2-4a and Table 2-1) that π_{GC} is identical to systemic-plasma oncotic pressure *only* at the very beginning of the glomerular

----

[2] Why the phrase "tend to" in this sentence? The basic equation relating K_f and GFR predicts that any decrease in K_f should definitely cause a directly proportional decrease in GFR. However, this prediction does not apply to GFR under conditions in which filtration pressure equilibrium occurs well before the end of the glomerular capillaries. The reason is that filtration, although reduced proportionally to K_f at every locus along the length of the capillary, will continue beyond the point in the capillary at which filtration pressure equilibrium previously had occurred. In this way, the total volume filtered along the entire length of the capillary may change little, if at all.

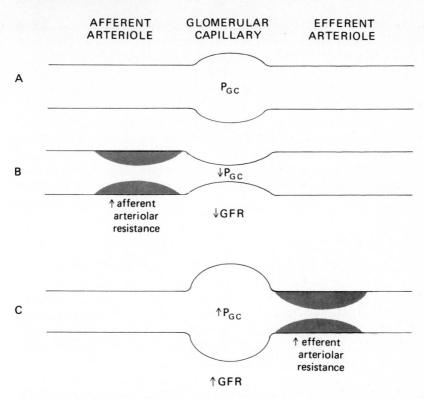

Figure 2-5 Effects of pure afferent- (B) or efferent- (C) arteriolar constriction on P_{GC} and, hence, GFR. See text for a qualification of the tendency for GFR to increase because of increased efferent-arteriolar constriction.

capillaries, and that π_{GC} then progressively increases along the glomerular capillaries as protein-free fluid filters out of the capillary, concentrating the protein left behind. As we have seen, this means that net filtration pressure and, hence, GFR progressively decrease along the capillary length. Accordingly, anything that favors a steeper rise in π_{GC} will tend to lower total GFR. This is what happens when total renal plasma flow is low—it shouldn't be hard to visualize that the initial filtration of a given volume of fluid from a small total volume of plasma flowing through the glomeruli will cause the protein left behind to become more concentrated than if the total volume of plasma were quite large. In other words, the presence of a low rate of total plasma flow through the glomeruli, all other factors being constant, will cause π_{GC} to rise more steeply. Thus, there exists the potential for an automatic link between total renal plasma flow and GFR, an increase or decrease in the former tending to cause an automatic change of similar direction in the latter. However, although conclusive data are not available, this automatic link between renal plasma flow and GFR is probably not a very important one, quantitatively, in human beings under most physiological conditions[3]; it was included here for the sake of completeness and will not be considered in subsequent chapters.

Summary   Table 2-2 presents a summary of the material described in this section. It provides, in essence, a check list of questions to ask when trying to ascertain why GFR has changed in any particular situation. First, which of the *direct* determinants of GFR is responsible for the change in GFR? Second, what factor is responsible for the change in this direct determinant? Finally, and not shown in the table, the normal physiological inputs (nerves, hormones, etc.) regulating these latter factors will be described in Chaps. 5 and 7.

TUBULAR REABSORPTION

Many filterable plasma components are either completely absent from the urine or present in smaller quantities than were originally filtered at the glomerulus. This fact alone is sufficient to prove that these substances undergo tubular reabsorption. An idea of the magnitude and importance of these reabsorptive mechanisms can be gained from Table 2-3, which summarizes data for a few plasma components, all of which are handled by filtration and reabsorption. These are typical values for a normal person on an average diet. There are at least three important conclusions to be drawn from this table: (1) The quantities of material entering the nephron via the glomerular filtrate are enormous, generally larger than their total body stores. If reabsorption of water ceased but filtration continued, the total plasma water would be urinated within 30 min. (2) The quantities of waste products, such as urea, which are excreted in the urine are generally sizable fractions of the filtered amounts. Thus, in mammals, coupling a larger glomerular filtration rate with a limited urea reabsorptive capacity permits rapid excretion of the large quantities of this substance produced constantly as a result of protein breakdown. (3) In contrast to urea and other waste products, the amount of most "useful" plasma components, e.g., water, electrolytes, and glucose, that are excreted in the urine represent quite small fractions of the filtered amounts. For this reason one often hears the generalization that the kidney performs its regulatory function by *completely* reabsorbing all of these biologically important materials and, thereby, preventing their loss from the body. This is a misleading half-truth, the refutation of which serves as an excellent opportunity for reviewing essential features of renal function and regulatory processes in general.

---

[3] The relationship is extremely important only in those species in which filtration pressure equilibrium occurs (see Suggested Readings for Chap. 2).

Table 2-3   Average Values for Several Substances Handled by
Filtration and Reabsorption

Substance	Amount filtered per day	Amount excreted	% reabsorbed
Water, L	180	1.8	99. 0
Sodium, g	630	3.2	99. 5
Glucose, g	180	0	100
Urea,*g	56	28	50

*Handling of urea is actually more complicated than just filtration and
reabsorption (see Chap. 4).

Let us begin by pointing out the part of the generalization that is true. Certain substances, notably glucose, are not normally excreted in the urine because the amounts filtered are completely reabsorbed by the tubules. But does such a system permit the kidneys to *regulate* the plasma concentration of glucose, i.e., *set* it at some specific concentration? The following example will point out why the answer is no. Suppose the plasma glucose concentration is 100 mg/100 mL. Since reabsorption of this carbohydrate is complete, no glucose is lost from the body via the urine, and the plasma concentration remains at 100 mg/100 mL. If, instead of 100 mg/100 mL, we set our hypothetical plasma glucose concentration at 60 mg/100 mL, the analysis does not change; no glucose is lost in the urine and the plasma glucose stays at 60 mg/100 mL. Obviously, the kidney is merely maintaining whatever plasma glucose concentration happens to exist and is not involved in the regulatory mechanisms by which the original setting of the plasma glucose was accomplished. It is not the kidney but primarily the liver and the endocrine system that set and regulate the plasma glucose concentration. [4] For comparison, consider what happens when a person drinks a lot of water: Within 1 to 2 h all the excess has been excreted in the urine, chiefly, as we shall see, as the result of decreased renal-tubular reabsorption of water. In this example, the kidney is the effector organ of a reflex that maintains plasma water concentration within very narrow limits. The critical point is that for many "useful" plasma components, particularly the inorganic ions and water, the kidney does *not completely* reabsorb the total amounts filtered. The rates at which these substances are reabsorbed (and, therefore, the rates at which they are excreted) are constantly subject to physiological

[4] Time and research give the lie to all generalizations. It is now known that the renal tubular cells actually *synthesize* glucose and release it into the blood during a prolonged fast. In this manner the kidneys do help set the plasma glucose concentration during prolonged fasting. This in no way detracts from the discussion above, which describes how glucose *reabsorption* does *not* contribute to the setting.

control. This ability to vary the reabsorption rates of water, sodium, calcium, phosphate, and many other substances (and to vary the secretion rates of still others) is really the essence of the kidney's ability to regulate the internal environment.

A bewildering variety of ions and molecules is found in the plasma and, therefore, in the glomerular filtrate, and most are reabsorbed to varying extents. It is essential to realize that tubular reabsorption is a qualitatively different process from glomerular filtration. The latter occurs by bulk flow, in which water and all dissolved free (non-protein-bound) crystalloids move together; this bulk flow occurs both because the appropriate net filtration pressure exists to drive it and because the glomerular wall has "pores" large enough to permit filtration. In contrast, there is relatively little bulk flow across the tubular-epithelial cells from lumen to interstitium because neither of these conditions is met; there are little, if any, hydraulic and oncotic pressure gradients, and the tubular epithelium is relatively much less porous than the glomerular membrane. (Recall that tubular-epithelial cells are joined together by tight junctions.) It must be emphasized that we are speaking here only of the relative lack of bulk flow from tubular lumen to interstitium; as will be discussed in Chap. 6, there is considerable bulk flow from interstitial fluid into peritubular capillaries, and this constitutes one of the ways (diffusion being the other) for a reabsorbed substance, having made it from tubular lumen to interstitial fluid, to complete its journey by gaining entry to the peritubular capillaries.

Given that bulk flow is not the important mechanism for transport of substances across the tubular-epithelial cells, it follows that tubular reabsorption of various substances is not by mass movement but rather by more or less discrete transport processes. The phrase "more or less discrete" denotes several important facts: (1) The reabsorption of different substances may be linked (for example, the reabsorption of many amino acids, glucose, and other solutes is linked to that of sodium); (2) a single reabsorptive system may be capable of transporting several distinct, but structurally similar, substances (for example, at least four of the simple carbohydrates are reabsorbed by a single system).

What are these transport mechanisms involved in tubular reabsorption? They are basically the same mechanisms involved in membrane transport anywhere in the body, and any discussion of transport is complicated by the problem of terminology.

Classification of Transport Mechanisms

Simple Diffusion   This process arises from random molecular motion and requires the presence of an electrochemical gradient for net movement to occur; i.e., net diffusion is always "downhill." Because simple diffusion proceeds mainly through the lipid matrix of the membrane, lipid solubility is a major determinant of any substance's diffusibility; only very small polar substances penetrate to any great extent by simple diffusion, presumably because they move through water-filled spaces trapped in the lipid matrix or water-filled "pores" created by the arrangement of the membrane's proteins. In contrast to the next four transport processes to be discussed, simple diffusion involves no specific interaction between the moving molecule and the proteins of the membrane.

Simple Facilitated Diffusion   This process, like simple diffusion, can produce net movement of a substance only down its electrochemical gradient (thus, the term "diffusion"). However, unlike simple diffusion, the transport is dependent upon interaction of the substance with specific membrane proteins, which "facilitate" its movement; therefore, the rate of movement is much higher than would be expected by simple diffusion (but net movement is still downhill). This is an important mechanism for accelerating the movement of non-lipid-soluble molecules, and the membrane proteins involved are termed either channels or carriers. A channel may be thought of as a pore, in that it penetrates the membrane, but it is formed by one or more proteins and has considerable specificity for the molecules or ions that move through it. The initial event in carrier-mediated facilitated diffusion is the binding of the molecule to be transported to the carrier, but the next events that lead to facilitation of the molecule's translocation across the membrane remain unknown. Because of the interaction with membrane proteins (whether channels or carriers), facilitated diffusion manifests specificity, saturability, and competition; none of these characteristics is exhibited by simple diffusion.

Secondary Active Transport   In this process, two (or sometimes more) substances interact simultaneously with the same specific membrane proteins (carriers), and both are translocated across the membrane. The crucial point is that one of the substances undergoes only net "downhill" transport (simple facilitated diffusion), whereas the other can manifest net "uphill" movement against its electrochemical gradient. Yet, the latter occurs without input of metabolic energy directly into the transport process. Rather, the direct source of energy in the process is the energy liberated by the simultaneous downhill facilitated diffusion of the other transported substance. In other words, as one of the substances (often sodium) moves down its electrochemical gradient, the energy released somehow is able to drive the other substance uphill against its electrochemical gradient. The substance moving uphill is said to undergo *secondary active transport* (the derivation of this term will become clear in a subsequent section).

The term *co-transport* denotes the situation in which the involved substances are moving in the same direction (one downhill and the other uphill). *Countertransport* is analagous to co-transport in that two or more substances interact simultaneously with the same specific membrane proteins and are translocated across the membrane; the difference is that the energy liberated by the downhill movement of one of the substances produces uphill movement of the second substance in the *opposite* direction (e.g., the downhill movement of sodium into the cell might provide the energy for uphill movement of hydrogen ion out of the cell).

Primary (Traditional) Active Transport   In this process, the transported molecule also interacts with membrane proteins (carriers) and may exhibit specificity, saturability, and competition. Its hallmark is net uphill transport, i.e., net transport against an electrochemical gradient, with the energy for this active transport coming *directly* from the splitting of ATP. Indeed, the term "primary" specifically denotes that metabolically produced chemical energy is the direct source of the energy for the process; in such cases, membrane-bound ATPase not only splits the ATP to provide energy but is a component of the actual carrier mechanism.

Endocytosis   This process is characterized by the invagination of a portion of the plasma membrane until it becomes completely pinched off and exists as an isolated intracellular membrane-bound vesicle filled with the extracellular fluid it imbibed during its formation. This process offers an important mechanism for the uptake of macromolecules, which may trigger off the entire process by binding to specific membrane proteins. Endocytosis, of course, requires energy, and its source is the splitting of ATP. Thus, endocytosis is technically a form of primary active transport.

Transport Mechanisms in Reabsorption

We began this discussion of tubular reabsorptive mechanisms with the statement that they are simply the basic mechanisms for tranport across any cell membranes, but we must now face the added complexity that arises when one deals with an epithelial layer, such as the renal tubule (or gastrointestinal epithelium, gallbladder epithelium, etc.), rather than the plasma membrane of a single nonepithelial cell (a muscle cell or erythrocyte, for example). The problem is quite straightforward (Fig. 2-6): Except for the few substances that are reabsorbed by simple diffusion across the tight junctions *between* cells, all other reabsorbed substances must cross *two* plasma membranes in their journey from tubular lumen to interstitial fluid—the *luminal (or apical) membrane* (separating the luminal fluid from the cell cytoplasm) and the *basolateral membrane* (separating the cytoplasm from

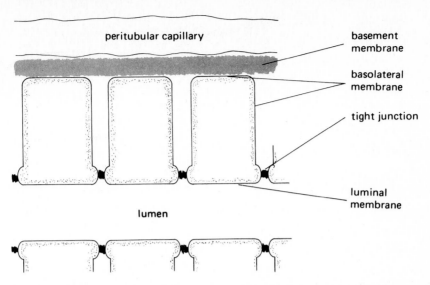

Figure 2-6 Diagrammatic representation of tubular epithelium. The tight junctions can be visualized three-dimensionally as the sheet of plastic holding together a six-pack of beer (each cell being one of the cans).

the interstitial fluid). (The basement membrane, upon which the epithelial layer rests (Fig. 2-6) must also be traversed, but because it serves only a structural role and is not a significant barrier to the movement of solutes or water, we shall ignore it; for this reason it will not be shown in subsequent figures illustrating either reabsorptive or secretory processes.) Accordingly, in order to fully characterize the overall transport of a substance across the epithelium, one must know what transport characteristics exist for the luminal membrane and the basolateral membrane.

Let us take sodium reabsorption as an example (Fig. 2-7). Sodium ions move across the luminal membrane into cytoplasm mainly by simple facilitated diffusion. They are then actively transported across the basolateral membrane into the interstitial fluid. This latter "pump" is a primary active process which involves Na-K-dependent ATPase, found only in the basolateral membranes. Finally, the sodium ions, along with water, move into the peritubular capillaries by bulk flow. (Bulk flow or simple diffusion into the peritubular capillaries is the final step in the reabsorption of all substances.) Thus, the unidirectional reabsorptive movement of sodium is made possible by the asymmetry of the luminal- and basolateral-membrane transport processes. What may not be apparent from this brief description is the fact that the luminal and basolateral events do not occur in isolation from each other. This becomes evident as soon as one recognizes that the continued net movement of sodium across the luminal membrane (being a simple facilitated diffusion process) depends completely upon the maintenance of a

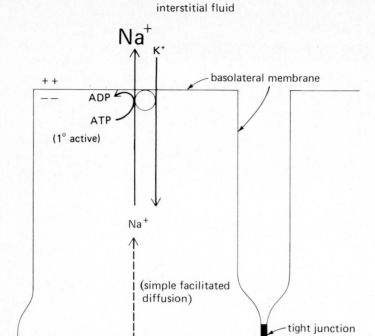

Figure 2-7 Reabsorption of sodium. Net facilitated diffusion into the cell is made possible by the low cytoplasmic [Na] and the potential difference, both ultimately the result of the basolateral primary active "pump." The fate of the potassium ions pumped into the cell by the Na-K-dependent ATPase is not shown in the figure so as to focus only on the sodium.

favorable electrochemical gradient — cytoplasmic [Na] < luminal [Na] and electric potential oriented so that the cell interior is negative relative to the lumen. The crucial point is that the basolateral Na-K-dependent ATPase pump creates this electrochemical gradient by keeping the cytoplasmic [Na] low and the cell interior negatively charged. (The exact role of the pump in the creation of intracellular negativity is not dealt with here.)

Let us take another example, the reabsorption of glucose (Fig. 2-8). Glucose moves from the lumen across the luminal membrane into the cytoplasm by secondary active transport coupled to the facilitated diffusion of sodium. (This carrier is quite distinct from the simple facilitated diffusion carrier used by most sodium ions; i.e., sodium moves into the cell by a variety of facilitated diffusion pathways.) The energy utilized to drive uphill movement of glucose across the luminal membrane is derived from the simultaneous downhill movement of sodium. So efficient is this uphill movement that the lumen can be virtually cleared of glucose. After entry into the cell, the glucose then exits across the basolateral membrane by simple facilitated diffusion, this downhill movement being driven by the high glucose concentration achieved in the cell by the action of the luminal transport process. A critical point, easy to miss, is that the entire overall process of glucose reabsorption depends ultimately upon the primary active sodium pump in the basolateral membrane! Only because of this pump is the electrochemical gradient maintained for net facilitated diffusion of sodium across the luminal membrane, and it is this downhill process that provides the energy for the simultaneous uphill movement of the glucose. Now the reader should be able to understand why glucose reabsorption is termed secondary active transport—it is itself uphill ("active") but is "secondary" to (dependent upon) "primary" active transport of sodium. Instead of glucose, we could have used amino acids, phosphate, or a variety of organic substances as our example, for they, too, undergo secondary active reabsorption by being co-transported with sodium in precisely the same manner.

Despite the breakdown of the traditional categorization of transport processes as simply "active" or "passive," renal physiologists still find it helpful to use these terms to characterize the overall reabsorptive process for any given substance. In such usage, "active" simply is a shorthand way of stating that at least one of the two membrane crossings is achieved by a primary or secondary active process, i.e., that uphill transport against the substance's electrochemical gradient has occurred somewhere between lumen and interstitial fluid. Thus, we say that glucose undergoes active reabsorption.

Transport Maximum

Many of the active reabsorptive systems in the renal tubule can transport only limited amounts of material per unit time, primarily because the membrane proteins responsible for the transport become saturated. The classical example is the transport process for glucose in the proximal tubule. As we have seen, normal persons do not excrete glucose in their urine because tubular reabsorption is complete. But it is possible to produce urinary excretion of glucose in a completely normal person merely by administering large quantities of glucose directly into a vein (Table 2-4).

Note that even after the plasma glucose concentration has doubled, the urine is still glucose-free, indicating that the *maximal tubular transport capacity (T_m)* for reabsorbing glucose has not yet been reached. But as the

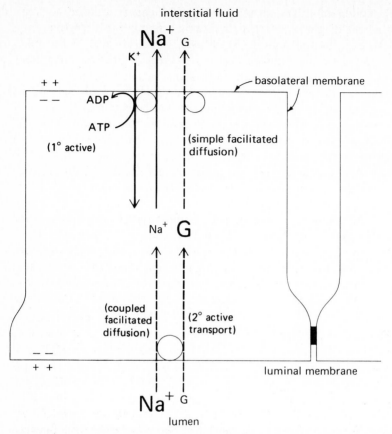

Figure 2-8 "Secondary active reabsorption" of glucose. Follow this figure by beginning with the primary active Na pump in the basolateral membrane. Then you will see how the low intracellular [Na] and intracellular negativity permit the net downhill entry of Na across the luminal membrane, which, in turn, provides the energy for simultaneous uphill glucose movement across this membrane. Luminal [glucose] is shown falling toward zero as it is reabsorbed.

plasma glucose and the filtered load continue to rise, glucose finally appears in the urine. From this point on, any further increase in plasma glucose is accompanied by a proportionate increase in excreted glucose because the T_m, which equals 375 mg/min, has now been reached. The tubules are now reabsorbing all the glucose they can, and any amount filtered in excess of this quantity cannot be reabsorbed and appears in the urine. This is precisely what occurs in patients with diabetes mellitus. Because of a deficiency in pancreatic production of insulin, the patient's plasma glucose may rise to extremely high values. The filtered load of glucose becomes great enough to exceed the T_m, and glucose appears in the urine. There

Table 2-4   Experimental Data Obtained for Calculation of Glucose T_m

Time, min	GFR, mL/min	P_G, mg/mL	Filtered glucose (GFR × P_G), mg/min	Excreted glucose ($U_G V$),* mg/min	Reabsorbed glucose (filtered − excreted), mg/min
0	125	1.0	125	0	125
Begin glucose infusion					
26–40	125	2.0	250	0	250
100–110	125	4.0	500	125	375
130–140	125	5.0	625	250	375

*U_G = urine concentration of glucose; V = urine volume per time.

is nothing wrong with the tubular transport mechanism for glucose. It is simply unable to reabsorb the huge filtered load.

To add one more level of complexity, let us return to the experiment in which glucose was infused. Additional data were obtained for minutes 60 to 100 but were not shown in Table 2-4. They are as follows:

Time, min	GFR, mL/min	P_G, mg/mL	Filtered glucose, mg/min	Excreted glucose, mg/min	Reabsorbed glucose, mg/min
60–80	125	2.8	350	20	330
80–100	125	3.5	436	76	360

Now we see that glucose began to be excreted in the urine *before* the true T_m of 375 mg/min was reached (the plasma concentration at which glucose first appears in the urine is known as the *threshold* for glucose). There are several reasons for this so-called *splay:* (1) A carrier-mediated mechanism shows kinetics analogous to those of enzyme systems so that maximal activity is substrate-dependent (in this case, glucose-dependent); i.e., the pump may not work at its absolute maximal rate until the luminal glucose concentration is too high to permit all of it to be "captured" by the pump. (2) Not all nephrons have the same T_m for glucose, so that some may be spilling glucose at a time when others have not yet reached their T_ms. This last point is extremely important, for we too often fall into the habit of viewing the kidneys as one large nephron. The fact is that there are really more than 2 million nephrons in the kidneys, and they are not identical in functional characteristics.

Except for our experimental subject receiving intravenous glucose, the plasma glucose in normal persons never becomes high enough to cause urinary excretion of glucose, because the reabsorptive capacity for glucose is much greater than necessary for normal filtered loads. However, for certain other substances, the reabsorptive T_m is very close to the normal filtered load (perhaps already in the splay portion of the reabsorptive pattern); therefore, even a small increase in the plasma concentration of such a substance would produce large increases in its excretion.

TUBULAR SECRETION

Tubular secretory processes, which transport substances across the tubular epithelium into the lumen (i.e., in the direction opposite to tubular reabsorption), constitute a second pathway into the tubule, the first pathway being glomerular filtration.

The overall secretory process for any given substance begins with its simple diffusion out of the peritubular capillaries into the interstitial fluid, from which it makes its way into the lumen by crossing either the tight junctions (in some cases of simple diffusion) or, in turn, the basolateral and luminal membranes of the cell. In the latter cases, the net unidirectional movement results from differences in the characteristics of the two membranes. For example (Fig. 2-9), the secreted substance might be pumped across the basolateral membrane by a primary or secondary active process and the resulting high intracellular concentration could then drive movement across the luminal membrane by facilitated diffusion. Of course, positioning of the active secretory step on the luminal membrane and the passive step on the basolateral membrane would achieve the same final result, i.e., net movement into the tubular lumen. As is true for tubular reabsorption, the overall process of tubular secretion can be categorized as active or passive depending upon whether an uphill process occurs at one or both membranes.

Since the first step in the active secretion of a substance is simple diffusion of the substance from peritubular capillary into interstitial fluid, one might suppose that substances mainly bound to plasma proteins could not undergo tubular secretion. However, such is not the case. There are always some free molecules of the substance in equilibrium with those bound to plasma proteins, and as the free molecules diffuse out of the capillary, others come off the plasma proteins by mass action to take their place. This happens rapidly enough so that, in those cases where a secretory system exists for a protein-bound substance, almost all of the substance originally bound to the protein can still undergo secretion, often during a single passage of blood through the kidneys.

Among the most important secretory processes are those for hydrogen ion and potassium, and these will be discussed in detail later. There also exist (in the proximal tubule) several low-specificity secretory systems for

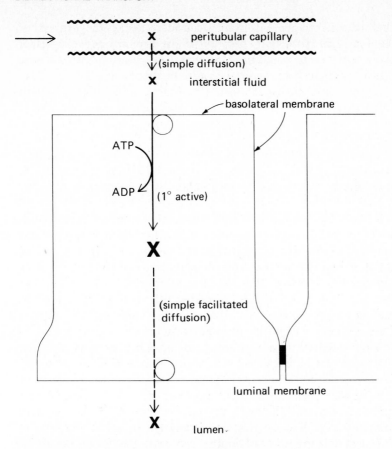

Figure 2-9 Secretory pathway for hypothetical substance X.

organic anions and cations (see Chap. 4). These are analogous to the proximal reabsorptive mechanism described above for glucose in that they are active, are T_m-limited, and manifest competition.

BIDIRECTIONAL TRANSPORT

In the preceding sections, the adjective "net" was frequently used in reference to tubular reabsorption or secretion and was always implicit even when absent. The fact is that only rarely, if ever, does any transported substance manifest purely unidirectional flux across the tubule totally unopposed by a flux in the other direction. One reason for this is that the epithelium is not completely impermeable to crystalloids, so that bidirectional diffusion is always occurring even in the absence of diffusion gradients.

Another reason is apparent from reconsideration of the example illustrated in Fig. 2-9. Note that, because of the primary active transport
process in the basolateral membrane, the overall secretory process achieves
a concentration gradient between lumen and interstitial fluid. This gradient,
of course, favors a net movement in the reabsorptive direction by simple
diffusion so that if the tight junctions or cell membranes themselves are at
all permeable to substance X, such movement will occur. Similarly, active
reabsorptive processes tend to establish a concentration gradient between
lumen and interstitial fluid that favors passive secretion. Thus, we are dealing with so-called pump-leak systems, in which the active "pump" creates
a diffusion gradient that opposes its own action by favoring back-diffusion.
Since this back-diffusion occurs solely as an indirect result of the pump's
activity and since the *net* flux will, therefore, always be in the direction
of the pump, we do not usually dignify the back-diffusion with the terms
reabsorption or secretion. In other words, in reference to Fig. 2-9, we say
simply that X is handled by secretion (and do not call the passive back-
flux "reabsorption"). To take the sodium pattern of Fig. 2-7 as another
example, we say simply that sodium is reabsorbed (and do not assign the
term "secretion" to the passive back-flux into the lumen secondary to the
concentration gradient created by the sodium pump).

The "leak" component of epithelial "pump-leak" systems is a very
important determinant of the maximal concentration gradients that can be
established across the epithelial layer. Thus, to refer again to Fig. 2-9, the
more permeable the epithelium is to X, the more difficult it will be for the
secretory mechanisms (the "pump") to increase luminal X concentration
above interstitial-fluid X concentration. Similarly, an active reabsorptive
mechanism is less able to lower the luminal concentration of the transported
substance below its interstitial-fluid concentration when the permeability
of the epithelial layer to that substance is very high.

For most mineral ions and many organic molecules, the major route
for passive diffusion (the "leak") is not "transcellular" (crossing both luminal and basolateral membranes) but rather "paracellular" (crossing the
junctional complexes between cells). On the basis of the relative permeability of the junctional complexes (and, hence, of the epithelial layer),
various epithelia are classified as "leaky" or "tight." Leaky epithelia include
the proximal tubules (as well as the epithelia of the small intestine and
gallbladder); tight epithelia include the distal tubules and collecting tubules.

To reiterate, leaky epithelia do not achieve large ionic concentration
gradients between lumen and interstitial fluid. In addition, only relatively
low electrical potentials exist across them (because the passive leak "short-
circuits" the potentials); they have high water permeabilities; and they
generally can actively transport large quantities of ions. In contrast, tight
epithelia exhibit large potential differences, low water permeabilities, and

relatively slow rates of active transport of ions; however, because of their low permeability to the back-leak of ions and water, these slow rates of active transport can achieve quite large concentration differences across the epithelium. These characteristics should be kept in mind when we discuss, in subsequent chapters, the transport of ions and water by the proximal (leaky) and distal (tight) segments of the tubule.

Pump-leak systems are not the only cause of bidirectional transport. Another reason is that a nephron segment may contain either distinct opposing pathways or "reversible pumps" for a single substance. This may seem strange, but such systems do exist, and the nephron segment may, therefore, manifest net secretion or net reabsorption depending upon the physiological circumstances.

Finally, for many substances, a given nephron segment may always manifest only reabsorption or only secretion, but other nephron segments may do just the opposite. For example, a substance may be secreted into the proximal tubule but reabsorbed from the distal tubule; in such cases, the relative magnitudes of the opposing processes in the different nephron segments determine whether the overall tubular effect will be reabsorption or secretion.

METABOLISM BY THE TUBULES

Although renal physiologists have traditionally listed glomerular filtration, tubular reabsorption, and tubular secretion as the three basic renal processes, a fourth fate — metabolism by the tubular cells — is also of considerable importance for many substances. For example, the cells may extract organic nutrients from the peritubular capillaries but rather than secreting them into the lumen, the cells may metabolize them as dictated by the cells' own nutrient requirements. In so doing, the renal cells are behaving no differently than any other cells in the body.

In contrast, other metabolic transformations performed by the kidney are not directed toward its own nutritional requirements but rather toward altering the composition of the urine and plasma. The most important of these are the synthesis of ammonia from glutamine, and the "synthesis" of bicarbonate, both described in Chap. 9.

Study questions: 3 to 12

CHAPTER 3

RENAL CLEARANCE

OBJECTIVES

The student understands the principles and applications of clearance technique.

1 Defines the term clearance
2 States which clearances are used to measure GFR and ERPF
3 Lists the data required for clearance calculation
4 Given data, calculates C_{In}, C_{PAH}, C_{urea}, $C_{glucose}$, C_{Na}
5 Predicts whether a substance undergoes net reabsorption or net secretion by comparison of its clearance to that of inulin, or by comparison of its rate of filtration to its rate of excretion
6 Given data, calculates net rate of reabsorption or secretion for any substance
7 Given data, calculates reabsorptive T_m for glucose and secretory T_m for PAH
8 Given data, calculates fractional excretion of any substance
9 Given data, uses the "double ratio" to determine whether a particular nephron segment reabsorbs or secretes a substance
10 Knows how to estimate GFR from C_{urea} and describes the limitations
11 Describes the limitation of C_{Cr} as a measure of GFR
12 Constructs the curve relating steady-state P_{Cr} to C_{Cr} or P_{urea} to C_{urea}; predicts the changes in P_{Cr} and P_{urea} given a known change in GFR; knows the limitations of this analysis, particularly with regard to urea

The technique known as *clearance* is extremely useful for evaluating renal function. Before defining it and developing it in a more formal manner, we will look at an example of how it is used—the measurement of glomerular filtration rate.

MEASUREMENT OF GFR

Assume there is a substance (let us call it W) that is freely filterable at the glomerulus but neither secreted nor reabsorbed by the tubules. Then:

$$\frac{\text{Mass of W excreted}}{\text{Time}} = \frac{\text{Mass of W filtered}}{\text{Time}} \tag{1}$$

Since the mass of any solute equals the product of solute concentration and solvent volume,

$$\frac{\text{Mass of W excreted}}{\text{Time}} = \frac{\text{Urine conc of W} \times \text{urine volume}}{\text{Time}} \tag{2}$$

Combining Eqs. (1) and (2):

$$U_W V = \frac{\text{Mass of W filtered}}{\text{Time}} \tag{3}$$

where U_W = urine concentration and V = urine volume per unit time.

Of course, the mass of W filtered also equals the product of the volume of plasma filtered into Bowman's capsule and the concentration of W per unit volume of filtrate. The volume of plasma filtered per unit time is, by definition, the *glomerular filtration rate* (GFR). Since W is freely filterable, the filtrate concentration of W is the same as the plasma concentration P_W. Therefore:

$$\frac{\text{Mass of W filtered}}{\text{Time}} = P_W \times \text{GFR} \tag{4}$$

Combining Eqs. (3) and (4):

$$U_W V = P_W \times \text{GFR} \tag{5}$$

Three of the variables — V, P_W, and U_W — can be measured, and we can solve for GFR:

$$\text{GFR} = \frac{U_W V}{P_W} \tag{6}$$

The validity of the above analysis depends upon the following characteristics of W:

    1 Freely filterable at the glomerulus
    2 Not reabsorbed
    3 Not secreted
    4 Not synthesized by the tubules
    5 Not broken down by the tubules

A polysaccharide called *inulin* (not insulin) completely fits this description and can be used for the determination of GFR. Consider the following hypothetical situation: In order to determine your patient's GFR, you infuse inulin at a rate sufficient to maintain plasma concentration constant at 4 mg/L. Urine collected over a 2-h period has a volume of 0.2 L and an inulin concentration of 360 mg/L. What is the patient's GFR?

$$\text{GFR} = \frac{U_{In}V}{P_{In}}$$

$$\text{GFR} = \frac{360 \text{ mg/L} \times 0.2 \text{ L/2 h}}{4 \text{ mg/L}}$$

$$\text{GFR} = 18 \text{ L/2 h} = 9 \text{ L/h}$$

If any of the five criteria listed above were not valid for inulin, its use would not provide an accurate measure of GFR. For example, if inulin were secreted, which of the following statements would be true?

    Calculated GFR would be higher than the true GFR.
    Calculated GFR would be lower than the true GFR.

    The first statement is correct because the mass of inulin excreted would represent both filtered and secreted inulin and, therefore, would be greater than the filtered inulin.
    Unfortunately, measuring GFR with inulin is inconvenient because inulin is not a normally occurring bodily substance and must, therefore, be administered intravenously at a continuous constant rate for several hours. Therefore, in clinical situations the endogenous substance *creatinine* is frequently used to *estimate* GFR. Creatinine is formed from muscle creatine and released into the blood at a fairly constant rate. Consequently, its blood concentration changes little during a 24-h period so that one need obtain only a single blood sample and a 24-h urine collection.

$$\text{Estimated GFR} = \frac{U_{Cr}V}{P_{Cr}}$$

This is only an estimated GFR because in humans, creatinine does not meet all five criteria; it is secreted by the tubules. It therefore overestimates the true GFR. However, the amount secreted is relatively small, and the discrepancy is not very large. In a later section we will describe how measurement of plasma creatinine alone without any urine determinations can also be used to estimate GFR more crudely. Use of urea for the same purpose will also be described.

DEFINITION OF CLEARANCE

When we described how inulin could be used to measure GFR, we were actually describing the technique known as clearance. First, let us define the term. The *clearance* of a substance is the *volume* of *plasma* from which that substance is *completely cleared* by the kidneys *per unit time*. Every substance in the blood has its own distinct clearance value, and the units are always in volume of plasma per time. Inulin offers an excellent first example. Since all excreted inulin must come from the plasma, one can see that a certain volume of plasma loses its inulin while flowing through the kidney; i.e., a certain volume of plasma is "cleared" of inulin. For inulin, this volume is obviously equal to the GFR, since none of the inulin contained in the glomerular filtrate returns to the blood (inulin is not reabsorbed) and since none of the plasma that escapes filtration loses any of its inulin (inulin is not secreted). Therefore, a volume of plasma equal to the GFR has been completely cleared of inulin. This volume is termed the inulin clearance and is expressed as C_{In}. Accordingly,

$$C_{\text{In}} = \text{GFR}$$

What is the glucose clearance? Glucose is freely filtered at the glomerulus so that all the glucose contained in the glomerular filtrate is lost *initially* from the plasma to the tubules. But, all of this filtered glucose is normally then reabsorbed; i.e., it is all returned to the plasma. The net result is that *no* plasma ends up losing glucose; the clearance of glucose is *zero*.

Let us take another example — phosphate (for the purposes of this example, we will assume that plasma phosphate, P_{PO4}, is completely filterable):

$$\text{GFR} = 180 \text{ L/day}$$
$$P_{\text{PO}_4} = 1 \text{ mmol/L}$$
$$U_{\text{PO}_4}V = 20 \text{ mmol/day}$$

What is the phosphate clearance in this example? The filtered phosphate equals 180 mmol/day. Is this the phosphate clearance? The answer is no. Clearance does *not* designate a filtered mass. Indeed, it does not designate any mass; it is always a volume per time. The clearance of phosphate is defined as the volume of plasma completely cleared of phosphate per unit time. Is the clearance of phosphate, then, the GFR? Again the answer is no. Certainly, the filtered phosphate contained in the GFR is *temporarily* lost from the plasma, but much of it is reabsorbed, in this example, 160 mmol/day, leaving only 20 mmol/day to be excreted in the urine. Is this the phosphate clearance?

Once again the answer is no. Clearance is not defined as mass excreted but rather as the volume of plasma supplying that mass per unit time. In other words, the phosphate clearance is the volume of plasma which supplies the excreted 20 mmol; it is this volume which is completely cleared of its phosphate. How much plasma has to be completely cleared of phosphate to supply the 20 mmol? We know from the data that the plasma phosphate concentration equals 1 mmol/L. Therefore, it would take

$$\frac{20 \text{ mmol/day}}{1 \text{ mmol/L}} = 20 \text{ L/day}$$

to supply the excreted phosphate. Clearance of a substance answers the question: How much plasma must be completely cleared to supply the excreted mass of that substance? $C_{PO4} = 20$ L/day.

BASIC FORMULA

It should be evident, therefore, that the basic clearance formula for any substance X is:

$$C_X = \frac{\text{mass of X excreted/time}}{P_X}$$

$$C_X = \frac{U_X V}{P_X}$$

where C_x = the clearance of substance X
$\quad\quad U_x$ = urine concentration of X
$\quad\quad V$ = urine volume per time
$\quad\quad P_x$ = arterial plasma concentration of X[1]

C_{In} is a measure of GFR simply because the volume of plasma completely cleared of inulin, i.e., the volume from which the excreted inulin comes, is equal to the volume of plasma filtered. C_{PO4} must be less than

---

[1] In performing clearances, limb-vein blood may be used rather than arterial blood as long as the substances being studied are not synthesized or metabolized by the tissues of the limb.

C_{In} because much of the filtered phosphate is reabsorbed; therefore, less plasma was cleared of phosphate than of inulin.

Thus, the following generalization emerges: Whenever the clearance of a freely filterable substance is less than the inulin clearance, tubular reabsorption of that substance must have occurred. This is simply another way of stating that whenever the mass of a substance excreted in the urine is less than the mass filtered during the same period of time, tubular reabsorption must have occurred. The phrase "freely filterable" is essential in the above generalization. Protein serves as an excellent example. The clearance of protein in a normal person is essentially zero, obviously lower than the C_{In}. However, this does not prove that protein is reabsorbed; the major reason for the zero clearance is that the protein is not filtered. Accordingly, in order to compare inulin clearance to the clearance of any completely or partially protein-bound substance (calcium, for example), one must use the filterable plasma concentration of the substance, rather than the total plasma concentration, in the clearance formula.

Is the clearance of creatinine in humans higher or lower than that of inulin? The answer is higher. Like inulin, creatinine is freely filtered and not reabsorbed; therefore, a volume of plasma equal to that of the GFR (i.e., the C_{In}) is completely cleared of creatinine. But, in addition, a small amount of creatinine is secreted. Therefore, some plasma in addition to that filtered is cleared of its creatinine by means of tubular secretion. The clearance formula is precisely the same as that for any other substance:

$$C_{Cr} = \frac{U_{Cr}V}{P_{Cr}}$$

Another generalization emerges: Whenever the clearance of a substance is greater than the inulin clearance, tubular secretion of that substance must have occurred. Again, this is merely another way of stating that whenever the excreted mass exceeds the filtered mass, secretion must be occurring.

Another substance secreted by the proximal tubules is the organic anion para-aminohippurate (PAH). PAH is also filtered at the glomerulus, and, when its plasma concentration is fairly low, virtually all the PAH that escapes filtration is secreted. Since PAH is not reabsorbed, the net effect is that all the plasma supplying the nephrons is completely cleared of PAH. If PAH were completely cleared from all the plasma flowing through the *entire* kidney, then its clearance would measure the *total renal plasma flow* (TRPF). However, about 10 to 15 percent of the total renal plasma flow supplies nonsecreting portions of the kidneys, such as peripelvic fat and the medulla, and this plasma cannot, therefore, lose its PAH by secretion. Accordingly, the PAH clearance actually measures the so-called *effective renal plasma flow* (ERPF) and is approximately 85 to 90 percent of the true *total* renal plasma flow. The clearance formula for PAH is, of course:

$$C_{PAH} = \frac{U_{PAH}V}{P_{PAH}} = ERPF$$

Once we have measured the ERPF,[2] we can calculate easily the *effective renal blood flow* (ERBF):

$$ERBF = \frac{ERPF}{1 - V_c}$$

where V_c = the blood hematocrit, i.e., the fraction of blood occupied by erythrocytes.

It should be emphasized that C_{PAH} measures ERPF only when plasma PAH is fairly low. If plasma PAH were increased to a level so high that the PAH secretory T_m were exceeded, then PAH would not be completely removed from the plasma, and the use of its clearance as a measure of ERPF would be invalid. Another substance that is handled in a manner similar to PAH is Diodrast; accordingly, C_D is also a measure of ERPF.

Urea clearance C_{urea} can be determined by the usual formula:

$$C_{urea} = \frac{U_{urea}V}{P_{urea}}$$

Urea, like inulin, is freely filterable, but approximately 50 percent of filtered urea is reabsorbed; therefore, C_{urea} will be 50 percent of C_{In}. If the mass of urea reabsorbed were always exactly 50 percent of that filtered, could C_{urea} be used to estimate GFR? The answer is yes. One would merely multiply the C_{urea} by 2 to obtain a value equal to the GFR. Unfortunately, as will be described in Chap. 4, urea reabsorption varies between 40 and 60 percent of the filtered urea so that one cannot merely multiply by 2.

---

[2] To reiterate, C_{PAH} measures ERPF not TRPF because some PAH escapes filtration and secretion. However, we can measure the amount that has escaped simply by measuring the concentration of PAH in the renal venous plasma. We can then measure TRPF by using this value in the following equation:

$$TRPF = \frac{U_{PAH}V}{arterial\ _{PAH} - renal\ venous\ _{PAH}}$$

It should be evident that this equation is simply another example of the law of conservation of mass: What comes in at the renal artery must go out by the renal vein and urine combined.

Nonetheless, the clearance is easy to perform clinically and can be used as at least a crude indicator of glomerular function. The creatinine clearance is certainly a better way of evaluating GFR. But recall that, because of creatinine secretion, it is not completely accurate either.

QUANTITATION OF TUBULAR REABSORPTION AND SECRETION USING CLEARANCE OR MICROPUNCTURE

To reiterate, once a method (determination of C_{In}) is available for measuring GFR, it becomes possible to determine whether the overall nephron manifests net reabsorption or net secretion of any given substance. If the clearance of the substance (using the filterable plasma concentration in the calculation) is less than that of inulin, net reabsorption must be occurring; if the clearance of the substance is greater than that of inulin, net secretion exists. Why the word "net" in the above statements? Because the finding that a substance's clearance is less than that of inulin definitely proves reabsorption but does not disprove secretion; secretion might also have been present but masked by a greater rate of reabsorption. Similarly, proof of the presence of overall secretion ($C_X > C_{In}$) does not disprove the possibility that reabsorption, too, is present but of lesser magnitude than secretion.

Calculation of the magnitude of the net reabsorption or secretion in units of mass per time is given for any substance by the following equation:

$$\text{Mass excreted} = \text{Mass filtered} + \text{Mass secreted} - \text{Mass reabsorbed}$$
$$(U_X V) \qquad (GFR \cdot P_X)$$
$$(C_{In} \cdot P_X)$$

Rearranging terms:

$$\text{Mass filtered} - \text{Mass excreted} = (\text{Mass reabsorbed} - \text{Mass secreted})$$
$$(C_{In} \cdot P_X) \qquad\quad (U_X V)$$

Note that reabsorption and secretion are not *directly measured* variables, but are derived as a single value from the measurements of filtered and excreted masses; a positive value (filtered > excreted) quantifies net reabsorption, and a negative value (filtered < excreted) net secretion. (We have previously used this type of quantitation several times without formally defining it; for example, in Chap. 2, for the calculation of glucose T_m.)

Another common way of quantitating the degree of net reabsorption or net secretion is as fractional excretion (FE). FE answers the question: What fraction of the filtered mass of a substance does the excreted mass represent?

$$\frac{\text{Mass excreted}}{\text{Mass filtered}} = \text{Fractional excretion}$$

$$\frac{U_X V}{\text{GFR} \times P_X} = \text{FE}_X$$

Thus an FE_X of 0.23 means that, overall, the mass of X excreted is 23 percent of the mass of X filtered; therefore 77 percent of the filtered X has undergone net reabsorption. An FE_X of 1.5 means that 50 percent more X is excreted than was filtered; i.e., secretion is occurring.

Note that when inulin is used to measure GFR, the formula for fractional excretion is simply the ratio of C_X/C_{In}:

$$\frac{U_X V / P_X}{U_{In} V / P_{In}} = \text{FE}_X$$

Moreover, since urine volume (V) is common to both clearances it is not even necessary to measure V to calculate a fractional excretion:

$$\frac{U_X/P_X}{U_{In}/P_{In}} = \text{FE}_X$$

An analagous double ratio is the key to evaluating, using micropuncture, not overall tubular function but the presence of net reabsorption or net secretion in individual nephron segments. Let us take the handling of a hypothetical substance Q by the proximal tubule as an example. A sample of fluid is collected from the end of the proximal tubule in an experimental animal given inulin, and its concentrations of Q and inulin are measured and compared to those of arterial plasma. The fraction of filtered Q remaining at the end of the proximal tubule is given by the ratio:

$$\frac{\text{Tubular fluid}_Q / \text{Plasma}_Q}{\text{Tubular fluid}_{In} / \text{Plasma}_{In}}$$

The value is found to be approximately 0.6; i.e., about 60 percent of the filtered Q remains at the end of the proximal tubule. This means that 40 percent of the filtered Q had been reabsorbed by the proximal tubule. To determine what the loop of Henle has done, a sample of fluid is collected from the very early distal tubule and the "double ratio" for it compared to that for the end of the proximal; it is found to be 1.1, compared to 0.6 for the late proximal, establishing that Q has been secreted into the loop.

Similarly, a late distal sample can be compared to the early distal one to evaluate the net contribution of the distal tubule.

PLASMA CREATININE AND UREA CONCENTRATION AS INDICATORS OF GFR CHANGES

As described previously, the creatinine clearance is a close approximation of the GFR and is, therefore, a valuable clinical determination.

$$C_{Cr} = \frac{U_{Cr}V}{P_{Cr}}$$

In practice, however, it is far more common to measure plasma creatinine alone and to use this as an *indicator* of GFR. This approach is justified by the fact that most excreted creatinine gains entry to the tubule by filtration. If we ignore the small amount secreted, there should be an excellent inverse correlation between plasma creatinine and GFR, as shown by the following example: A normal person's plasma creatinine is 10 mg/L. It remains stable because each day the amount of creatinine produced is excreted. One day the GFR suddenly decreases permanently by 50 percent because of a blood clot in the renal artery. On that day the person filters only 50 percent as much creatinine as normal so that creatinine excretion is also reduced by 50 percent. (We are ignoring the small contribution of secreted creatinine.) Therefore, assuming no change in creatinine production, he or she goes into positive creatinine balance, and the plasma creatinine rises. But despite the persistent 50 percent GFR reduction, the plasma creatinine does not continue to rise indefinitely; rather, it stabilizes at 20 mg/L, i.e., after it has doubled. At this point the person once again is able to excrete creatinine at the normal rate and so remains stable. The reason is that the 50 percent GFR reduction has been counterbalanced by the increase in plasma creatinine, and filtered creatinine is again normal.

$$
\begin{aligned}
\text{Original normal state: Filtered creatinine} &= 10 \text{ mg/L} \times 180 \text{ L/day} \\
&= 1800 \text{ mg/day} \\
\text{New steady state:} \quad \text{Filtered creatinine} &= 20 \text{ mg/L} \times 90 \text{ L/day} \\
&= 1800 \text{ mg/day}
\end{aligned}
$$

What if the GFR then fell to 30 L/day? Again creatinine retention would occur until a new steady state had been established, i.e., until the person

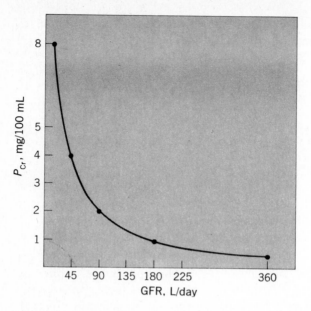

Figure 3-1 Steady-state relationship between GFR and plasma creatinine (assuming no creatinine is secreted).

is again filtering 1800 mg/day. What would the new plasma creatinine be?

$$1800 \text{ mg/day} = P_{Cr} \times 30 \text{ L/day}$$
$$P_{Cr} = 60 \text{ mg/L}$$

It should now be clear why a single plasma creatinine is a reasonable indicator of GFR (Fig. 3-1). It is not completely accurate for three reasons: (1) Some creatinine is secreted. (2) There is no way of knowing exactly what the person's original creatinine was when GFR was normal. (3) Creatinine production may not remain completely unchanged.

Since urea is also handled by filtration, the same type of analysis would indicate that the measurement of plasma urea concentration could serve as an indicator of GFR. However, it is a much less accurate indicator than plasma creatinine because the range of normal plasma urea concentration varies widely, depending upon protein intake and changes in tissue catabolism, and because urea is reabsorbed to a *variable* degree. (The fact that it is reabsorbed would not interfere with its use as an indicator if the reabsorption were always a *fixed* percent of the filtered mass.)

Study questions: 13 to 23

CHAPTER 4

RENAL HANDLING OF ORGANIC SUBSTANCES

OBJECTIVES

Student understands the renal handling of certain organic substances.

1 States the major characteristics of the proximal-tubular systems for reabsorption of organic nutrients
2 Describes the renal handling of proteins
3 Describes the renal handling of urea
4 Describes the proximal secretory system for organic anions; describes the overall renal handling of PAH
5 Describes the renal handling of urate
6 Describes the proximal secretory system for organic cations
7 Describes, in general terms, the renal handling of weak acids and bases, including the contributions of glomerular filtration, active proximal secretion, and passive movements secondary to water reabsorption or pH changes; given any change in luminal pH, predicts the change in net transtubular movement for a substance with a particular pK.

All subsequent chapters of this book will deal almost exclusively with the renal handling of inorganic substances, since regulation of their excretion constitutes the kidneys' major physiological role. However, as pointed out in Chap. 1, another major renal function is the excretion of organic waste products, foreign chemicals, and their metabolites. Moreover, reabsorptive processes must exist to prevent massive excretion of filtered organic nutrients. An analysis of the renal transport pathways for all these organic substances is well beyond the scope of this book, but this chapter briefly describes certain of the major ones.

GLUCOSE, AMINO ACIDS, ET AL.; PROXIMAL REABSORP-
TION OF ORGANIC NUTRIENTS

The proximal tubule is the major site of reabsorption of the large quantities of organic nutrients filtered each day by the glomeruli. These include glucose, amino acids, several Krebs cycle intermediates, certain water-soluble vitamins, lactate, acetoacetate, β-hydroxybutyrate, and still others. The characteristics of glucose reabsorption described in examples used earlier in Chap. 2 are typical of the transport processes for most (but not all) of them:

   1 They are active in that they can reabsorb their respective solutes against electrochemical gradients. Indeed the intraluminal concentration of the substance can often be reduced virtually to zero. Such marked transtubular concentration gradients can be established for these organic nutrients because there is only a modest "leak" of the molecules from the interstitial fluid back into the lumen across the tight junctions between cells. (The statement made in a previous chapter that the proximal tubule is "leaky" and, hence, unable to achieve large concentration gradients was with regard to inorganic ions, not organic solutes.)

   2 The "uphill" step is across the luminal membrane, usually via co-transport with sodium. Movement across the basolateral membrane from cell into interstitium is simple facilitated diffusion.[1]

   3 They manifest T_ms which are usually well above the amounts *normally* filtered; accordingly, the kidneys protect against loss of the substances but do not help set their plasma concentrations. However, as we saw for glucose in diabetic persons, under abnormal conditions, the plasma concentration of any of these substances may become so increased as to cause the reabsorptive T_m for it to be exceeded and large quantities to be lost in the urine. Good examples are acetoacetate and β-hydroxybutyrate in patients with severe uncontrolled diabetes.

   4 They manifest specificity. This means that there are a large number of different "carriers" (i.e., membrane proteins with which the different solute types interact). But there is by no means a one-to-one correspondence, since two or more closely related substances may utilize the same carrier. For example, the amino acid reabsorptive mechanisms are quite distinct from those for glucose (and other monosaccharides), but there are not 20 separate processes (one for each amino acid); rather there is one for

---

[1] For some amino acids "uphill" transport from interstitial fluid into cell, i.e., in the direction opposite the reabsorptive movement, has been demonstrated. Presence of this carrier explains why, under certain circumstances, net secretion, rather than net reabsorption, of these amino acids occurs. The physiological significance of this secretion is not known.

arginine, lysine, and ornithine; another for glutamate and aspartate; and so on. The existence of shared pathways allows for competition among those substances utilizing any given pathway; for example, the administration of large quantities of ornithine partially blocks the reabsorption of the other amino acids that share its pathway. (This is, of course, explainable on the basis of competition for the common carrier's binding sites.)

5 They are inhibitable by a variety of drugs and diseases. There are persons with genetic defects manifested as a deficit in one or more of these proximal reabsorptive systems (so-called inborn errors of transport). In some cases, the deficit may be highly specific (involving only one amino acid, for example), whereas in others, multiple systems may be involved (glucose and many amino acids, for example). This range of defects is also seen when the deficit is due to an external agent rather than to a genetic abnormality.

PROTEINS AND PEPTIDES

The proximal tubule is also the major site for protein reabsorption, but it is listed separately here to emphasize its importance and the fact that its reabsorptive pathway is quite different from those for the substances listed in the preceding section. As mentioned above, there is a very small amount of protein in the glomerular filtrate. The normal concentration approximates 10 mg/L, about 0.02 percent of plasma albumin concentration. Yet this is *not* negligible because of the huge volume of fluid filtered per day.

$$\text{Total filtered protein} = \text{GFR} \times \text{filtrate conc of protein}$$
$$= 180 \text{ L/day} \times 10 \text{ mg/L}$$
$$= 1.8 \text{ g/day}$$

If none of this protein were reabsorbed, the entire 1.8 g would be lost in the urine. In fact, virtually all of the filtered protein is reabsorbed so that the excretion of protein in the urine is normally only 100 mg/day. The mechanism by which protein is reabsorbed is easily saturated, so any large increase in filtered protein resulting from increased glomerular permeability can cause the excretion of large quantities of protein. For example, suppose that disease causes the glomeruli to allow 1 percent of the plasma albumin to be filtered:

$$\text{Filtered albumin} = \text{GFR} \times (50 \text{ g/L}) \ (0.01)$$
$$= 180 \text{ L/day} \times 0.5 \text{ g/L}$$
$$= 90 \text{ g/day}$$

This is far greater than the reabsorptive T_m for protein, and large quantities of albumin would be lost in the urine.

The initial step in protein reabsorption is endocytosis at the luminal membrane. This energy-requiring process is triggered by the binding of filtered protein molecules to specific sites on the luminal membranes; therefore, the rate of endocytosis is increased in proportion to the concentration of protein in the glomerular filtrate until a maximal rate of vesicle formation (and, thus, the T_m for protein reabsorption) is reached. The pinched-off intracellular vesicles resulting from endocytosis merge with lysosomes, whose enzymes degrade the protein to low-molecular-weight fragments (mainly individual amino acids). These end products are then released across the basolateral membrane into the interstitial fluid, from which they gain entry to the peritubular capillaries. It should be evident from this description that the term *reabsorption*, in reference to protein handling, is unusual, since the intact protein molecules themselves are not actually being moved from lumen to interstitial fluid but are catabolized in the renal tubular cells. (There may be a small number that actually do make the trip, since a few intact endocytotic vesicles move through the cell cytoplasm and empty their proteins by exocytosis into the interstitial fluid.) Nevertheless, the important point is that the filtered protein is not excreted in the urine and is, in this sense, reabsorbed.

Discussions of renal handling of protein logically tend to focus on albumin, since it is by far the major plasma protein, quantitatively. There are, of course, many other plasma proteins and it should be reemphasized here that many of these proteins, being smaller than albumin, are filtered to a greater degree. For example, growth hormone (m.w. = 20,000) is approximately 60 percent filterable. This means that relatively large fractions of these smaller plasma proteins are filtered at the glomeruli and degraded in tubular cells; accordingly, the kidneys are major sites of catabolism of many plasma proteins.

Finally, smaller linear polypeptides (such as angiotensin) are handled quite differently from proteins. They are completely filterable at the glomerulus, and are then catabolized, mainly into amino acids, within the proximal tubular lumen by peptidases located on the luminal plasma membrane; the amino acids as well as very small peptides generated by this process are then reabsorbed.

UREA

Just as glucose provides an excellent example of an actively transported solute, urea (the primary end product of protein catabolism) provides an example of transport by simple diffusion. Urea is a highly diffusible substance so that net movement across most biological membranes requires only the creation of a diffusion gradient for it. Such gradients exist within the kidneys, as the following analysis shows.

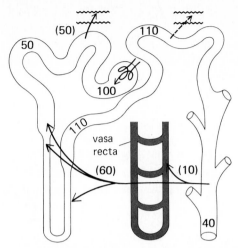

Figure 4-1 Renal handling of urea. The numbers in parentheses denote the percentages of filtered urea present at various sites along the tubule. It is not clear whether most of the secreted urea enters the straight portions of the proximal tubules or the descending and/or ascending thin limbs of the loop of Henle. (*Redrawn from H. Valtin, Renal Function: Mechanisms Preserving Fluid and Solute Balance in Health, Little, Brown, Boston, 1973.*)

Since urea is freely filtered at the glomerulus, its concentration in Bowman's capsule is identical to its concentration in peritubular-capillary plasma. Then, as the fluid flows along the proximal convoluted tubule, water reabsorption occurs, increasing the concentration of any intratubular solute not being reabsorbed at the same rate as the water. As a result, the concentration of urea in the tubular lumen becomes greater than the concentration of urea in the peritubular plasma. Accordingly, urea is able to diffuse passively down this concentration gradient from tubular lumen to interstitial fluid, and then into peritubular capillaries. Urea reabsorption is, thus, a passive process and completely dependent upon water reabsorption, which establishes the diffusion gradient.

Beyond the proximal convoluted tubule, the story becomes much more complicated. Let us pick up the fluid at the end of the proximal convoluted tubule, at which point approximately 50 percent of the urea has been reabsorbed, and follow it the rest of the way, using Fig. 4-1 as reference.

What happens in the straight portion of the proximal tubule and the loop of Henle? One might logically have predicted that more urea would be reabsorbed along with the water reabsorbed from these nephron segments (water reabsorption by the loop is described in Chap. 6), but such turns out not to be the case. By the beginning of the distal tubule, there is actually twice as much urea in the tubular fluid as originally left the proximal convoluted tubule (i.e., about the same amount as originally filtered)! Thus, *secretion* of urea into the straight portion of the proximal tubule and/or the loop of Henle has occurred. (For simplicity, the rest of this discussion will include the straight portion of the proximal tubule as part of the loop of Henle; it is not clear which of these segments participates to the greatest degree in urea secretion.) However, the source of this secreted urea is *not* peritubular plasma (the usual source of secreted solutes) and is best ignored for the present until we complete the tubular fluid's journey through the nephron.

Some of this enlarged amount of urea is reabsorbed (again by simple diffusion down its concentration gradient) in the distal tubule and cortical collecting tubule, but not much because these nephron segments are not very permeable to it. Therefore, most of the urea that entered the distal tubule from the loop drains into the medullary collecting tubules. There, particularly in the inner medulla, passive urea reabsorption once again becomes quite large both because of a high tubular permeability to urea and because of the extensive water reabsorption there. The urea which escapes reabsorption by the medullary collecting tubules amounts to approximately 40 percent of the amount originally filtered, and this is the urea excreted into the final urine. Thus, the *overall net* renal tubular handling of urea is the reabsorption of approximately 60 percent.

Now we can back up and point out the source of the urea that entered the loop of Henle by secretion — it is most of the urea that is reabsorbed by the collecting tubules. As illustrated in Fig. 4-1, as urea diffuses out of the collecting ducts into the interstitial fluid, the urea concentration of this fluid is raised, thereby creating a gradient for net diffusion of urea into the loops of Henle.

Thus, most of the urea that diffuses *out of* the collecting tubules (reabsorption) diffuses *into* the loops (secretion) and once more flows through the distal nephron, only to suffer the same fate again in the collecting tubules. In other words, a large quantity of urea is simply recycled between these segments of the nephron. Not all the urea that diffuses out of the collecting tubules is recycled in this manner, since some enters the medullary capillaries and is carried out of the kidneys.

In summary (Fig. 2-5), the renal handling of filtered urea is by simple diffusion.[2] Approximately 50 percent is reabsorbed into the blood across the proximal convoluted tubule. The remaining 50 percent undergoes a recycling sequence beyond the proximal convoluted tubule characterized by reabsorption out of the collecting tubules followed by secretion into the loop of Henle. Approximately 10 percent of the filtered urea escapes this recycling and makes it into the capillaries and back into the systemic circulation. The net result is that approximately 60 percent (50 percent by

---

[2] It is possible that some component of *active* reabsorption and/or secretion also exists along with these dominant passive components (see Suggested Readings for Chap. 3).

Table 4-1 Some Organic Anions Actively Secreted by
the Proximal Tubule

Endogenous Substances	Drugs
Bile salts	Acetazolamide
Fatty acids	Chlorothiazide
Hippurates	Ethacrynate
Hydroxybenzoates	Furosemide
Oxalate	Penicillin
Prostaglandins	Probenecid
Urate	Saccharin
	Salicylates
	Sulfonamides

the proximal and 10 percent by the rest of the nephron) of the filtered urea is truly (in the sense of "irrevocably") reabsorbed. This figure of 60 percent reabsorbed applies to situations in which the urine flow is relatively low (i.e., water reabsorption high). Only about 40 percent of the filtered urea is reabsorbed when the urine flow is high (i.e., water reabsorption low). This is because the diffusion gradient for urea reabsorption is created by water reabsorption, and the less the latter, the less will be the former.

To reiterate, the net reabsorption of filtered urea ranges between 40 and 60 percent. A crucial fact is that this same range applies regardless of how high the plasma urea concentration may be. Thus, urea reabsorption manifests no true T_m, in absolute terms, because it is governed by simple diffusion gradients and requires no interaction with membrane binding sites.

PAH, URATE, ET AL: PROXIMAL SECRETION OF ORGANIC ANIONS

The proximal tubule actively secretes a large number of different organic anions, both foreign and endogenously produced (see Table 4-1 for a partial listing). Many of the organic anions handled by this system are also filterable at the glomerulus, and so the amount secreted proximally adds to that which gains entry to the tubule via glomerular filtration. Others, however, are extensively bound to plasma proteins, and so undergo glomerular filtration only to a limited extent; accordingly, proximal-tubular secretion constitutes the only significant mechanism for their excretion (recall from Chap. 2 that binding to plasma proteins does not generally impede tubular secretion).

The active secretory pathway for organic anions in the proximal tubule has a relatively low specificity; i.e., a single system (or possibly several very closely related ones) is responsible for the secretion of all the organic anions listed in Table 4-1 and many more. The relatively nondiscriminating nature of this sytem accounts for its ability to eliminate from the body so many drugs and other foreign environmental chemicals. In this regard the liver's metabolic transformations are frequently important; in the liver, many foreign (and endogenous) substances are conjugated with either glucuronate or sulfate, and these two types of conjugates are actively transported by the organic-anion secretory pathway.

Perhaps the most intensively studied organic anion secreted by this pathway is the para-amino derivative of hippurate (PAH), since this substance, as we saw in Chap. 3, is used for the measurement of effective renal plasma flow. PAH is actively transported into proximal tubular cells across the basolateral membrane; the resulting high intracellular concentration then provides the gradient for the facilitated diffusion of PAH across the luminal membrane into the tubular lumen. (Thus, the pathway is similar to that previously shown for hypothetical substance X in Figure 2-4, but with one qualification: It is not known whether the basolateral entry step represents a primary active process or, as is more likely, a secondary active process — co-transport or countertransport with an inorganic ion.)

This mechanism for PAH secretion is shared by the other organic anions secreted proximally; i.e., they all share the same carriers. As might be predicted, there is competition for transport among these anions; i.e., an elevated plasma concentration of one of the substances will tend to inhibit the secretion of the others (thus, drugs used deliberately to inhibit proximal organic-anion secretion are usually, themselves, organic anions secreted by it). Another characteristic of this secretory system is T_m limitation: As the plasma concentration of an anion secreted by the system increases, so does the rate of secretion, until the transport maximum for that substance is reached, beyond which no further increase in secretion occurs. This direct relationship between plasma concentration and rate of secretion (at values below T_m) provides a simple but effective mechanism for homeostatically regulating the endogenous organic anions handled by the system and for speeding the excretion of foreign anions.

PAH is typical, in yet another way, of many (but not all) of the organic anions secreted proximally: It undergoes no significant tubular reabsorption anywhere along the nephron. Accordingly, the mass of PAH excreted per unit time is equal to the sum of the masses filtered (PAH is not protein-bound) and secreted.

In contrast, some of the organic anions secreted proximally can undergo significant passive tubular reabsorption, mainly in distal nephron segments, and the mechanisms of this passive reabsorption will be described in the last section of this chapter.

Finally, there are a few proximally secreted organic anions that also undergo active tubular reabsorption, mainly in the proximal tubule. The most notable example is urate. The major form of uric acid in plasma (and all but the most acid urines) is ionized urate. Urate is not protein-

Table 4-2 Some Organic Cations Actively Secreted by the Proximal Tubule

Endogenous Substances	Drugs
Acetylcholine	Atropine
Choline	Isoproterenol
Creatinine	Cimetidine
Dopamine	Meperidine
Epinephrine	Morphine
Guanidine	Procaine
Histamine	Quinine
Serotonin	Tetraethyl ammonium
Norepinephrine	
Thiamine	

bound and so is freely filterable at the glomerulus. Urate undergoes tubular reabsorption and tubular secretion; both are active processes, and both occur mainly in the proximal tubule. The rate of tubular reabsorption is normally much greater than the rate of tubular secretion; therefore, the net tubular effect is to remove urate from the lumen, and this explains why, in normal persons, the mass of urate excreted per unit time is only a small fraction of the mass filtered. However, although urate reabsorption is more extensive than secretion, it seems to be the rate of the secretory process that is homeostatically controlled to maintain relative constancy of plasma urate. In other words, if plasma urate begins to increase because of increased urate production, the rate of active proximal secretion of urate is stimulated, thereby increasing urate excretion. Many persons have elevated plasma concentrations of urate because they secrete and, hence, excrete less of this substance at any given plasma urate concentration than do normal persons. Other causes of renally induced elevations of plasma urate are decreased filtration of urate (due to decreased GFR) or excessive reabsorption of urate.

PROXIMAL SECRETION OF ORGANIC CATIONS

Proximal tubules possess an active-transport system (or several closely related systems) for organic cations that is quite analogous to that for organic anions: It is relatively nonspecific in that it transports a large number of foreign and endogenously occurring substances (Table 4-2) that compete with each other for transport, and it manifests a T_m limitation.

As is true for the proximal secretion of organic anions, that for organic cations is particularly critical for the excretion of those substances extensively bound to plasma proteins and not filterable at the glomerulus.

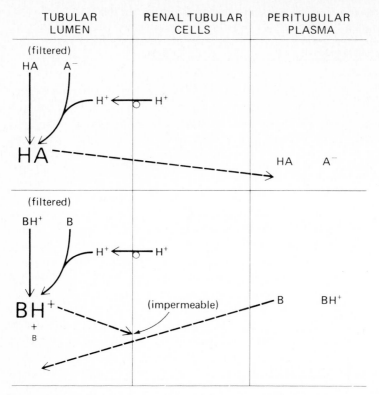

TUBULAR LUMEN	RENAL TUBULAR CELLS	PERITUBULAR PLASMA

Figure 4-2 Acidification of the luminal fluid creates, by mass action, the gradients which drive net passive reabsorption (→) of weak acids (top) and net passive secretion (←) of weak bases (bottom).

However, again similar to the case for the organic anions, many of the organic cations secreted by the proximal tubules are not protein-bound; creatinine is a good example.

Finally, and again analagous to the story for organic anions, some organic cations are not only actively secreted by the proximal tubules but may undergo other forms of tubular handling, mainly passive reabsorption or secretion, a subject to which we now turn.

PASSIVE REABSORPTION OR SECRETION OF WEAK ORGANIC ACIDS AND BASES

Many organic anions and cations are the ionized forms of weak acids and bases. Quite apart from any active tubular handling (mainly the proximal secretion described above), such substances (in their nonionized forms) may also undergo passive reabsorption or passive secretion, depending upon several conditions, the most important being the pH of the urine. To be specific, many weak acids undergo net tubular secretion when the urine is highly alkaline but net tubular reabsorption when it is acidic. The opposite pattern is seen for many weak organic bases.

To understand what accounts for this pH dependency, one must realize that the renal tubular epithelium, like other biological membranes, is mainly a lipid barrier; accordingly, highly lipid-soluble substances can penetrate it fairly readily by simple diffusion. Recall that one of the major determinants of lipid solubility is the polarity of a molecule; the more polar, the less lipid-soluble. Now, a weak acid exists as a polar ion in alkaline solution and as a nonpolar molecule in acid solution (the exact pH dependency of this reaction depends, of course, on the pK of the molecules in question):

$$A^- + H^+ \rightleftharpoons AH$$

For weak bases, the ionic form is favored in acid solutions.

$$B + H^+ \rightleftharpoons BH^+$$

Accordingly, the diffusible form of weak acids is generated in acidic fluid, whereas the diffusible form of weak bases is generated in alkaline fluid.

Let us now apply these principles using aspirin as an example and ignoring, for the moment, active proximal secretion of aspirin:

$$\underset{\text{(acetylsalicylate)}}{ASA^-} + H^+ \rightleftharpoons \underset{\text{(acetylsalicylic acid)}}{ASA\text{-}H}$$

Aspirin is filterable at the glomerulus, and so its concentration in Bowman's space is identical to that in peritubular plasma; moreover, because the pH of the glomerular filtrate is identical to that of peritubular plasma, the relative proportions of ASA$^-$ and ASA-H are also the same in the two fluids. As the filtered fluid flows along the tubule, water is reabsorbed, and this removal of solvent concentrates both ASA$^-$ and ASA-H, thereby creating lumen-to-plasma diffusion gradients favoring net reabsorption (exactly as described for urea). Since only ASA-H can penetrate the membrane to any great extent, only this form is reabsorbed. Simultaneously (and this is really the crucial point) secretion of hydrogen ions into the lumen lowers the luminal pH and favors, by mass action, the generation of ASA-H, which can then diffuse along its concentration gradient from lumen to peritubular plasma (Fig. 4-2). In other words, water reabsorption is one factor which helps create the concentration gradient required for passive reabsorption, but luminal acidification, by generating the diffusible form of the substance from the nondiffusible form, is even more important in creating the gradient.

But the story is even more interesting, for as we shall see in Chap. 9, the tubular fluid can be made alkaline rather than more acid under certain circumstances. This would shift the intraluminal reaction toward generation of ASA⁻ at the expense of ASA-H, and the resulting decrease in luminal ASA-H would, of course, reduce the gradient for net reabsorption. Indeed, luminal ASA-H might actually fall below peritubular-capillary plasma ASA-H, thereby establishing a gradient for net passive *secretion* of ASA-H rather than reabsorption. Thus, the net passive reabsorption of weak organic acids is inversely related to urine pH, and net passive secretion may be seen when the urine is alkaline.

We have been dealing only qualitatively with these concepts. The quantitative relationship is determined by the pK of the acid and the pH of the tubular fluid; for example, an acid with a pK well below the lowest tubular-fluid pH achievable—4.4—would exist within in the tubule mainly in the anionic (nondiffusible) form and thus always undergo relatively little passive reabsorption. In contrast, an acid with a pK of 6 would exhibit a marked increase in the degree of passive reabsorption if intratubular-fluid pH were lowered from 7 to 5, since the nonionized (diffusible) form would go from 10 percent of the total to 90 percent.

Readers should have little difficulty applying these same concepts to the passive renal tubular handling of weak bases: When the tubular fluid is highly acidic, the generation of BH$^+$ from B is favored; the BH$^+$ cannot diffuse out of the lumen because of its charge, but the lowering of intraluminal B favors net passive secretion of B from peritubular-capillary plasma into the lumen. Conversely, when the urine is alkaline, generation of B within the lumen is favored, and a gradient is established for net passive reabsorption. Thus, weak bases are reabsorbed passively when the urine is alkaline but may be passively secreted when it is acid. Because pH changes are, as we shall see, greatest in the more distal tubular segments, these segments are the major sites for such pH-dependent passive transport.

It must be reemphasized that the description in this section has been in terms only of *passive* reabsorption and secretion of these substances. The fact is, as described earlier in this chapter, *active* secretory mechanisms also exist in the proximal tubule for the anionic and cationic forms of many weak acids and bases. Accordingly, these forms may be actively secreted into the proximal-tubular lumen followed by either passive reabsorption or passive secretion of the nonionized forms there and in the subsequent nephron segments, depending in part on urine flow rate but mainly upon the change in luminal pH occurring along the tubule.

In summary, the excretion of a weak acid or base reflects the following factors:

1 The amount filtered at the glomerulus, which is determined by the product of the GFR and the ultrafilterable (non-protein-bound) plasma concentration of the substance.

2 The amount secreted actively by the proximal tubules; this increases with increasing plasma concentration until the T_m for that substance is reached. It is also sensitive to inhibition by competing anions.

3 The amount passively reabsorbed or secreted; this reflects the urine flow, the pK of the substance, and the pH of the urine.

Because so many medically used drugs are weak organic acids and bases, all these factors have important chemical implications. For example, if one wished to enhance the excretion of a drug that is a weak acid, one would attempt to alkalinize the urine; in contrast, acidification of the urine is desirable if one wished to prevent excretion of the drug. Of course, exactly the opposite would apply to weak organic bases. Increasing the urine flow would increase the excretion of both weak acids and bases. Finally, excretion could be reduced by giving another drug that interferes with any active proximal secretory pathway for the drug.

Study questions: 24 to 27

CHAPTER 5

CONTROL OF RENAL HEMODYNAMICS

OBJECTIVES

The student understands the control of renal hemodynamics.

1   States the formula relating flow, pressure, and resistance

2   Knows the normal rates of the GFR and RBF and defines filtration fraction

3   Defines autoregulation of RBF and GFR; states the condition in which "pure" autoregulation can be observed; states its adaptive function

4   Describes the myogenic and tubulo-glomerular feedback concepts to explain autoregulation

5   States how tubulo-glomerular feedback lowers GFR when proximal and/or loop reabsorption is inhibited

6   Describes the role of the renal sympathetic nerves and states when their activity is increased, including extrarenal baroreceptor reflexes

7   Describes how changes in filtration fraction occur

8   States the effect of angiotensin II on renal arterioles and glomerular mesangial cells

9   Describes the four major controls of renin secretion; identifies the type of adrenergic receptor involved in the direct sympathetic pathway

10   States the adaptive value of the renal vasoconstriction induced by the renal nerves and angiotensin II

11   States the effect of the renal nerves and angiotensin II on renal prostaglandin synthesis and the function served by the prostaglandins

12   States the effect of antidiuretic hormone on renal arterioles

13   Defines distribution of flow (cortex-medulla and cortex-cortex)

The total blood flow to the kidneys in a typical adult is approximately 1.1 L/min. Thus, the kidneys receive 20 to 25 percent of the total cardiac output (5L/min) even though their combined weight is less than 1 percent of total body weight! Given a normal hematocrit of 0.45, the total renal plasma flow = 0.55 × 1.1 L/min = 605 mL/min. Recall that the GFR equals 125 mL/min. Therefore, of the 605 mL of plasma that enters the glomeruli via the afferent arterioles, 125/605, or 20 percent, filters into Bowman's capsule, the remaining 480 mL passing via the efferent arterioles into the peritubular capillaries. This ratio is known as the *filtration fraction.*

The basic equation for blood flow through any organ is

$$\text{Organ blood flow} = \frac{\Delta P}{R}$$

where ΔP = mean arterial pressure minus venous pressure for that organ

R = resistance to flow through that organ

Recall that, normally, the major determinant of resistance is the radii of the arterioles within that organ, itself determined mainly by the degree of contraction of the arteriolar smooth muscle. It should be evident, therefore, that renal blood flow is determined mainly by the mean arterial pressure and the contractile state of the renal arteriolar smooth muscle.

MEAN ARTERIAL PRESSURE AND AUTOREGULATION

The renal circulation manifests quite markedly the phenomenon of *autoregulation*: The rate of blood flow through the kidney is relatively constant in the face of changes in mean renal arterial pressure—at least in the face of mean arterial pressures that range between 80 and 180 mmHg (Fig. 5-1). Look again at the basic cardiovascular equation above. This equation predicts that if the pressure gradient is increased by 50 percent and resistance stays constant, blood flow will increase 50 percent. In the kidney, however, such is not the case. If one isolates a kidney experimentally and perfuses it with blood by means of a pump, one can demonstrate that a 50 percent increase in pressure gradient produces less than a 10 percent increase in blood flow. There is only one possible explanation: Resistance in the kidney does *not* stay constant as arterial pressure increases. Rather, resistance automatically increases. The smooth muscle of the renal arterioles contracts to a greater degree, thereby decreasing the radii of the arterioles and, hence, increasing arteriolar resistance; therefore, blood flow remains relatively unchanged despite the increased arterial pressure.

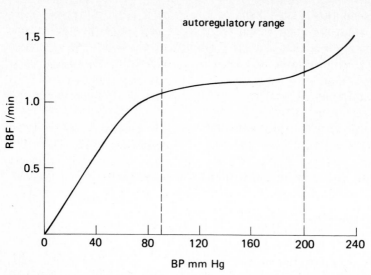

Figure 5-1 Autoregulation of renal blood flow (RBF). A similar pattern holds for glomerular filtration rate.

This entire discussion applies not only to RBF but to GFR, which also shows only small changes in the face of large changes in arterial pressure. There are several reasons for the fact the GFR, as well as RBF, is autoregulated. One of the most important is that the *afferent* arterioles are the major site of autoregulatory resistance changes in the face of arterial-pressure changes; accordingly, glomerular-capillary pressure (and, therefore, net filtration pressure) remains relatively unchanged.[1] For example, a rise in renal arterial pressure triggers enhanced afferent-arteriolar constriction, thereby increasing the pressure drop between the arteries and glomerular capillaries and preventing the transmission of the increased arterial pressure to the glomerular capillaries.

What is the mechanism of autoregulation; i.e., how does an increase in renal arterial pressure elicit enhanced contraction of the smooth muscle of renal arterioles, whereas a reduction in pressure elicits relaxation? One thing is for certain—the mechanism is completely intrarenal since it can be elicited in an isolated kidney perfused *in vitro*. There are two intrarenal mechanisms presently thought to be responsible for autoregulation: (1) a so-called *myogenic mechanism;* and (2) *tubulo-glomerular feedback.*

The myogenic mechanism is similar to that found in other (nonrenal) autoregulating vascular beds: Vascular smooth muscle actively contracts in response to increased stretch. Accordingly, an increased intra-arteriolar

---

[1] A second reason under certain circumstances is the automatic link between RBF and GFR described in Chap. 2.

pressure distends the arteriolar wall, i.e., increases its passive tension, and the inherent response of the smooth muscle in the wall is to contract, thereby increasing the resistance offered by the vessel. It is likely that the link between increased stretching of the wall and increased contraction is that the stretch opens plasma-membrane calcium channels, and, hence, permits increased flow of calcium across the plasma membrane into the cytosol of the smooth muscle cell.

Tubulo-glomerular feedback is a more complex process, which regulates GFR primarily, with changes of RBF being a secondary consequence. The basic pathway is illustrated in Fig. 5-2. An increased arterial pressure tends to raise glomerular-capillary pressure (P_{GC}) and RBF. The increase in P_{GC} raises GFR and, hence, the rate of fluid flow through the proximal tubule, loop of Henle, and macula densa. The macula densa cells (and/or possibly tubular cells distal to the macula densa) somehow detect the increased flow past them, and this triggers the generation of a vasoconstrictor chemical by one of the cell types in the juxtaglomerular apparatus (JGA). This vasoconstrictor acts on the smooth muscle of the adjacent arterioles (particularly the afferent arterioles) and causes vasoconstriction. The result is an increased afferent-arteriolar resistance, which decreases P_{GC} and, hence, GFR,[2] as well as RBF, i.e., counteracts the increases caused by the elevated renal arterial pressure.

A great deal remains unknown about tubulo-glomerular feedback. First, how does the macula densa detect changes in rate of fluid flow? It is known that increased fluid flow through the loop of Henle and into the macula densa is associated with increased luminal concentrations of sodium, chloride, and total solute (osmolarity), and one of these may be the variable detected (this will be covered in more detail in Chap. 7 in another context, the control of renin release). Second, what is the vasoconstrictor involved? It is likely that angiotensin II and prostaglandins play permissive roles, but are not the primary mediators. Adenosine (which constricts renal arterioles, in contrast to its vasodilator effect on most other vascular beds) is a possibility, but conclusive evidence is still lacking.

The examples used to illustrate the myogenic and tubulo-glomerular mechanisms employed *increases* in renal arterial pressures as the initial event. It should be clear, however, that, since mean arterial pressure is normally above the lower limit of the autoregulatory range (80 to 180 mmHg), *decreases* in arterial pressure will also be offset by the autoregulatory mechanisms: Decreased stretch of afferent-arteriolar smooth muscle causes

---

[2] A decrease in P_{GC} may not be the only reason that GFR decreases. Some evidence suggests that the vasoconstrictor released by the JGA acts not only upon the arterioles but on the glomerular mesangium as well; as described earlier, contraction of these mesangial cells would reduce the surface area of the glomeruli, thereby decreasing the filtration coefficient (K_f).

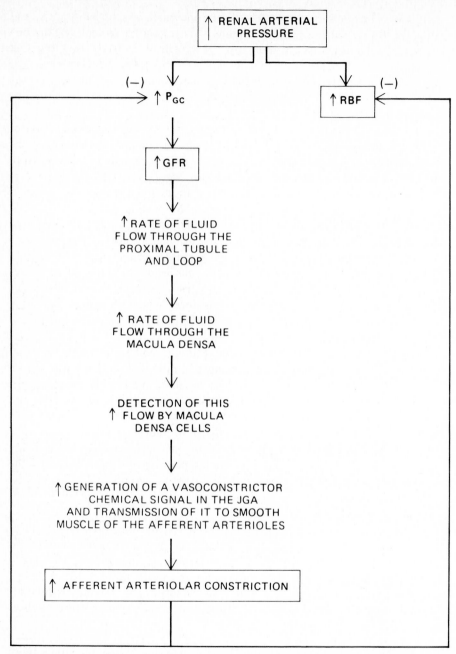

Figure 5-2 Tubulo-glomerular feedback contribution to autoregulation.

relaxation, i.e., less contraction, and decreased flow through the macula densa causes less of the relevant vasoconstrictor to be produced by the JGA. However, tubulo-glomerular feedback seems to be of lesser importance in this lower autoregulatory range.

What is the adaptive value of autoregulation? As in any other organ, it helps ameliorate blood-flow changes in the face of arterial-pressure fluctuations, but it also serves a unique role in the kidney, namely the blunting of the large changes in solute and water excretion which could otherwise occur because of large changes in GFR whenever arterial pressure changed. This is the adaptive value of GFR autoregulation. Recall that the normal net filtration pressure in the glomeruli is only about 17 mmHg. Accordingly, even relatively minor changes in arterial pressure could cause marked increases or decreases, in turn, of glomerular-capillary pressure, GFR, and solute and water excretion, were the changes not effectively blunted by automatically elicited changes in afferent-arteriolar tonus.

In this regard, it should be emphasized that although tubulo-glomerular feedback was introduced in the context of autoregulation, this pathway may be of greater importance in situations characterized not by changes in arterial pressure but rather by disease- or drug-induced blockade of fluid reabsorption in the proximal tubule or loop of Henle. Under such conditions, the resulting increase in macula densa flow will trigger, via the usual sequence of events, a decrease in GFR, and thereby limit the urinary loss of salt and water resulting from the defect in reabsorption. Note that, in these cases, tubulo-glomerular feedback actually causes GFR to go below normal, whereas during autoregulatory responses, it keeps GFR from going above normal.

Having pointed out the value of autoregulation, we must now emphasize three facts: (1) Autoregulation is not perfect. RBF and GFR *do change* when renal arterial pressure is changed, but they change to a much smaller degree than they would if autoregulation did not exist. (2) Autoregulation is virtually absent at mean arterial pressures below 70 mmHg and, therefore, cannot blunt GFR and RBF changes below this point. (3) Despite autoregulation, RBF and GFR *can be altered considerably*, even when the arterial pressure is within the autoregulatory range, by the factors to be described next—the sympathetic nervous system, the renin-angiotensin system, and prostaglandins.

SYMPATHETIC CONTROL

In the above discussion of autoregulation, we set up artificial experimental conditions in which renal blood pressure was changed without altering blood pressure in the other arteries of the body (an analogue of this in a person might be the presence of an obstruction in a renal artery). In order to demonstrate autoregulation clearly, this is necessary because, when the systemic arterial pressure decreases in the *intact* organism, neuroendocrine variables are brought into play. One of these variables is increased activity in the renal sympathetic nerves (and increased circulating epinephrine) reflexly mediated via the carotid sinus and aortic arch baroreceptors (Fig. 5-3). This sympathetic input causes renal afferent and efferent arteriolar constriction (via alpha-adrenergic receptors), which decreases RBF (there are also some beta-adrenergic receptors on renal arteriolar smooth muscle, but so few in comparison to the alpha-adrenergic receptors that epinephrine causes only vasoconstriction in the kidneys). Thus, although autoregulation blunts the *direct* effects on the kidney of changes in arterial pressure, *sympathetic reflexes* can cause changes in renal hemodynamics when systemic arterial pressure is altered.

A second fact is that GFR also decreases, although not to the same extent as RBF. The major reason for the decrease in GFR during enhanced sympathetic outflow to the kidneys is the increase in afferent-arteriolar constriction induced by this input (afferent-arteriolar constriction → increased afferent-arteriolar resistance → decreased glomerular-capillary hydraulic pressure → decreased GFR).

If sympathetic input were solely to the afferent arteriole, the decreases in GFR and RBF induced by increased sympathetic tone would be approximately proportional. However, both afferent and efferent arterioles receive sympathetic innervation and are constricted (though not necessarily to the same degree) when sympathetic tone is increased; therefore, GFR tends not to decrease as much as RBF. As described in Chap. 2, the reason for this is that, because the efferent arterioles lie beyond the glomerulus, an increase in their resistance tends to *raise* glomerular-capillary pressure — just the opposite of the effect of afferent-arteriolar constriction (Fig. 5-4). In other words, sympathetically induced afferent and efferent constriction induce opposing effects on glomerular-capillary pressure and, hence, GFR, but additive effects on total renal resistance and, hence, RBF.

Because GFR decreases relatively less than RBF, the GFR/RBF ratio increases. We shall make use of this fact in Chap. 7, when the control of salt and water excretion is described.

What is the adaptive value of this sympathetically mediated renal vasoconstriction triggered by a decrease in systemic arterial blood pressure? For one thing, it is simply a component of the rapidly occurring general homeostatic regulation of arterial pressure. The renal vasoconstriction contributes to a rise in total peripheral resistance, which helps rapidly restore the arterial blood pressure toward normal. But there is a second, less obvious, way in which renal vasoconstriction helps raise arterial pressure: lowering the excretion of sodium and water. We shall see in Chap. 7 that

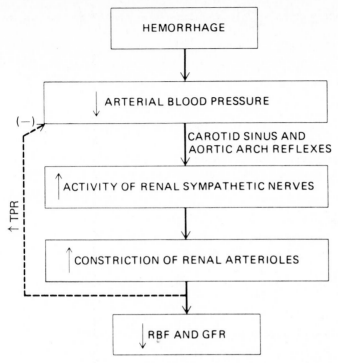

Figure 5-3 Pathway by which hypotension causes vasoconstriction mediated by the renal sympathetic nerves. Epinephrine, released from the adrenal medulla, also enhances renal vasoconstriction. The increased renal resistance helps to restore blood pressure (the negative-feedback loop) by contributing to increased total peripheral resistance (TPR).

this has important consequences for regulation of blood volume and, hence, arterial pressure. Renal vasoconstriction achieves a reduction in salt and water excretion both by lowering GFR (and, hence, the filtered load of these substances) and, as we shall see in Chap. 7, by increasing tubular reabsorption of these substances.

Finally, it should be emphasized that although this entire discussion has been in terms of the renal response to *arterial* hypotension, the same type of sympathetically mediated vasoconstriction can also be triggered by baroreceptors in the veins or cardiac chambers; indeed input from these baroreceptors probably has greater reflex effects on the renal circulation than does input from the arterial baroreceptors. Input from the peripheral chemoreceptors (responding to hypoxia) or from higher brain centers (for example, during heavy exercise or emotional situations) also can trigger increased sympathetic outflow to the kidneys.

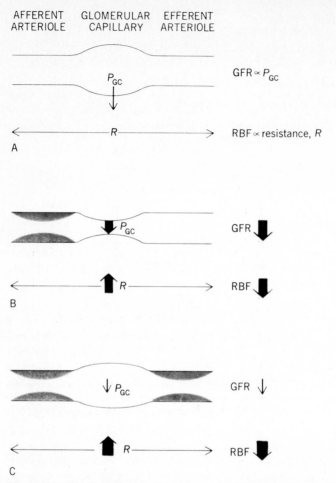

AFFERENT   GLOMERULAR   EFFERENT
ARTERIOLE   CAPILLARY   ARTERIOLE

P_{GC} $GFR \propto P_{GC}$

R $RBF \propto$ resistance, R

A

P_{GC} GFR

R RBF

B

$\downarrow P_{GC}$ GFR $\downarrow$

R RBF

C

Figure 5-4 Effects of afferent–(B) and combined afferent-efferent–(C) arteriolar constriction on GFR and RBF. Adding efferent constriction lowers RBF still further (because total resistance is increased) but restores GFR toward normal. The ratio GFR/RBF is, therefore, increased.

ANGIOTENSIN II

A second major regulator of the renal circulation is the renin-angiotensin system. Angiotensin II is a powerful vasoconstrictor, and the renal arterioles are quite sensitive to it. This hormone, like norepinephrine and epinephrine, constricts efferent arterioles as well as afferent arterioles,[3] and therefore also

[3] Although there is considerable controversy over whether angiotensin II exerts any effect at all on afferent arterioles, I believe the evidence favors the conclusion that this hormone normally does act on both sets of arterioles.

produces a lesser decrease in GFR than RBF (accordingly, the GFR/RBF ratio increases).

In addition to these actions on renal arterioles, angiotensin II causes contraction of glomerular mesangial cells, which results in a decrease in K_f, an additional factor contributing to a decrease in GFR. As described in Chap. 1, the plasma concentration of angiotensin II is increased when the kidneys are stimulated to secrete more renin; accordingly, angiotensin-induced renal vasoconstriction can be expected whenever renin secretion is significantly elevated.

Control of Renin Secretion

At this point, the student should review the basic biochemistry of the renin-angiotensin system and the anatomy of the juxtaglomerular apparatus, both described in Chap. 1. The control of renin secretion is quite complex, since there are at least four major types of inputs, which are strongly interrelated with one another.[4] These four mechanisms are (1) an intrarenal baroreceptor, (2) a tubular sodium (or chloride) receptor in the macula densa, (3) the renal sympathetic nerves, and (4) angiotensin itself.

Intrarenal Baroreceptors   The renin-secreting granular cells themselves act as baroreceptors (i.e., as pressure or distention receptors) monitoring the pressure or vascular volume within the last portions of the afferent arterioles (Fig. 1-3) and varying their secretion of renin inversely with these parameters. This makes good sense teleologically. For example, consider the response to hemorrhage: The pressure at the juxtaglomerular ends of the afferent arterioles is reduced both because of decreased arterial pressure and because of reflexly increased sympathetic outflow to the arterioles (Fig 5-3); the decreased arteriolar pressure would cause increased release of renin from the granular cells (Fig. 5-5).

Macula Densa   Earlier in this chapter, we described how the macula densa might be involved in tubulo-glomerular feedback—one of the mechanisms involved in autoregulation of GFR. Now we describe here another hypothesized function for the macula densa—control of renin secretion (some investigators believe that the tubulo-glomerular feedback and renin-control functions of the macula densa are one and the same, i.e., that the renin-angiotensin system is responsible for tubulo-glomerular feedback; on the basis of present evidence, this is unlikely).

---

[4] Despite the complexity, there is probably a final common pathway for all inputs controlling renin release—cytosolic calcium concentration. An increased cytosolic calcium concentration in the granular cells (or possibly, one of the other JGA cell types) inhibits renin release, whereas a decreased calcium concentration stimulates it. See Suggested Readings.

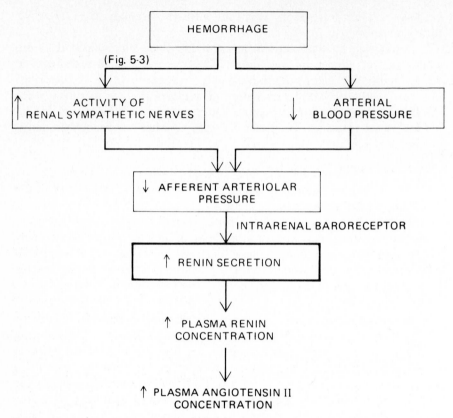

Figure 5-5 Intrarenal baroreceptor control of renin secretion during hemorrhage.

Because of the close anatomic relationship between the granular cells and the macula densa (Fig. 1-7), it is tempting to postulate that the renin-secreting granular cells are controlled, in part, by input from the macula densa concerning the composition of the fluid at the end of the ascending loop of Henle. Experimental evidence suggests that this is, indeed, the case. Specifically, the evidence suggests that renin secretion is *inversely* related to the mass of sodium chloride flowing into the macula densa: It is hypothesized that the actual signal is related not to the sodium chloride in the lumen of the macula densa but rather to the sodium or chloride concentration of the macula densa cells themselves. In this view, the rate of sodium chloride uptake by the cells is presumably proportional to the mass flowing by them; therefore, the sodium and chloride concentrations of the cell change in proportion to the load in the macula densa, and these changes somehow result in the generation of a chemical signal transmitted to the adjacent granular cells. The signal is inhibitory when the cell concentrations are high and stimulatory when low; whether sodium or chloride is the critical ion is not certain.[5]

Such a reflex makes sense teleologically, since it is simply a logical extension of the reflex described for the intrarenal-baroreceptor theory (Fig. 5-6).

Renal Sympathetic Nerves   We have already described one important mechanism by which an increased renal-sympathetic-nerve activity (and increased circulating epinephrine) result in an increase of renin secretion: by causing constriction of the afferent arterioles (Fig. 5-4). This stimulates the intrarenal baroreceptor by reducing the hydrostatic pressure at the end of the afferent arteriole, and it also stimulates the macula densa receptor by reducing the sodium load leaving the loop of Henle. In this manner, the renal sympathetic nerves play an important *indirect* role in controlling renin secretion.

In addition, sympathetic neurons end in the immediate vicinity of the granular cells (Fig. 1-7), and these neurons exert a *direct* stimulatory effect on renin secretion via beta-adrenergic receptors (most likely beta$_1$) on the granular cells. Actually, this direct effect is more sensitive than the indirect one involving renal vasoconstriction, since increases in sympathetic outflow to the kidneys too small to elicit vasoconstriction still cause increased renin secretion. This is preventable by drugs that block beta-adrenergic receptors.

Angiotensin II   Angiotensin II exerts a direct inhibitory effect on renin secretion by the granular cells. This is an example of a negative-feedback loop in which a hormone inhibits the secretion of its own stimulating substance, analogous to the inhibition of ACTH secretion by cortisol or to inhibition of TSH secretion by thyroxin. By this mechanism, angiotensin II exerts a dampening effect upon its own rate of production.

Other Inputs Controlling Renin Release   There are many inputs other than the four just described which have been shown to be capable of altering renin release; these include, among others, ADH, potassium, and calcium (all of which can inhibit renin release). The physiological significance of these pathways is mainly that they provide additional loops in the feedback mechanisms integrating the metabolism of sodium with that of water and other ions. Under most circumstances, they are of only minor importance, but this may not be true in clinical situations characterized by a large excess or deficit of any of them.[6]

Of particular interest is yet another input — renal prostaglandins. Several of the prostaglandins produced within the kidneys (notably PGE_2 and PGI_2)

---

[5] The entire question of the stimulus detected by the macula densa regarding renin secretion remains very controversial. Indeed, at least one investigator has postulated precisely the reverse of the entire hypothesis just described. (See Davis, 1973, Suggested Readings for Chap. 7, for a review of this field.)

[6] See Davis, 1973, in Suggested Readings.

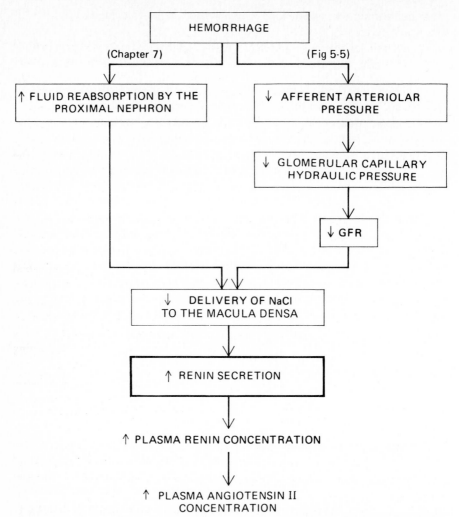

Figure 5-6 Macula densa control of renin secretion during hemorrhage. The pathway leading to decreased GFR is merely a continuation of Fig. 5-5. The mechanisms by which hemorrhage enhances fluid reabsorption by the proximal nephron will be described in Chap. 7.

can stimulate renin secretion, and these prostaglandins act as mediators or modulators of certain of the other inputs.[7]

---

[7] Present evidence suggests that beta-adrenergic control over renin secretion is independent of prostaglandins, but that the prostaglandins are somehow involved in, although probably not absolutely essential for, the macula densa and intrarenal-baroreceptor pathways.

PROSTAGLANDINS

We have just seen that the prostaglandins can exert an *indirect* control over the renal circulation via their participation in renin-releasing mechanisms. But, of greater importance are the *direct* effects of these potent vasoactive agents on the renal vasculature. Several of the renally produced prostaglandins (again notably PGE_2 and PGI_2) are vasodilators (particularly of the afferent arterioles), and the best documented physiological role for these vasodilator prostaglandins is to dampen the vasoconstrictor effect of the renal nerves and angiotensin II. An increased activity of the renal nerves or an increased plasma angiotensin II stimulates the kidney to synthesize and release vasodilator prostaglandins; the end result is that much of the vasoconstrictor actions of norepinephrine and angiotensin II are counteracted by the vasodilator action of the prostaglandins, and the renal resistance changes much less than would otherwise have occurred.[8]

Thus, if we return once more to our example of hypotension due to hemorrhage (Fig. 5-7), we see that three factors are reducing renal blood flow (and GFR) — the decreased blood pressure per se, the renal sympathetic nerves (and circulating epinephrine), and angiotensin II. Simultaneously, two factors are minimizing the reduction — autoregulation and the prostaglandins whose release is stimulated by the renal nerves and angiotensin II. The net result is usually a modest increase in renal vascular resistance, leading to a modest decrease in RBF (and GFR). The adaptive value of having such opposing inputs is to strike a balance between, on the one hand, the requirement for an increased total peripheral resistance to maintain systemic arterial pressure (for the "benefit" of the heart and brain) and, on the other hand, the likelihood of renal damage were renal vasoconstriction too severe. For example, an experimental animal given a drug that blocks prostaglandin synthesis and then subjected to even a modest hemorrhage may suffer rapid severe renal damage due to a profound reduction in renal blood flow.

The kidneys also produce several vasoconstrictor prostaglandins (notably TXA_2). No physiological role has yet been demonstrated for these vasoconstrictors. However, certain disease states (for example, ureteral obstruction and drug-induced acute renal failure) are associated with an increased intrarenal production of TXA_2 which may be a major cause of the intense and harmful vasoconstriction seen in these states.

---

[8] If one puts the information in this and the previous section together, it is apparent that a potential positive feedback mechanism exists between prostaglandins and the renin-angiotensin system: ↑renin release → ↑[renin] → ↑[angiotensin II] → ↑PG release → ↑[PG] → ↑renin release → etc. Whether such a positive feedback mechanism does, in fact, ever occur will remain unclear until we know more about the exact identities and sites of production of the various prostaglandins that interact with the renin-angiotensin system.

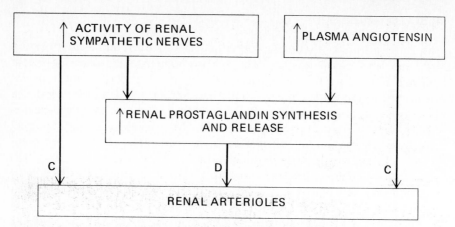

Figure 5-7 "Dampening" effect of prostaglandins on renal vasoconstriction induced by the renal nerves or angiotensin II (C = constriction; D = dilation).

OTHER FACTORS

The renal vasculature is sensitive to many other naturally occurring chemical messengers. Antidiuretic hormone (vasopressin), for example, causes renal vasoconstriction when present in high plasma concentrations. Dopamine is a renal vasodilator, and there is some evidence for the existence of renal-sympathetic-dopaminergic neurons. The intrarenally produced kinins (Chap. 1) are potent vasodilators, and adenosine (mentioned earlier as a possible mediator for tubulo-glomerular feedback) is a renal vasoconstrictor. However, whether dopamine, the kinins, and adenosine actually play significant roles in the control of renal hemodynamics remains to be determined.

INTRARENAL DISTRIBUTION OF BLOOD FLOW

Total renal blood flow can be measured readily either by clearance techniques or by more direct methods, such as flow probes. However, measurement of *regional* blood flows within the kidney has proven to be quite difficult. One well-established fact is that the cortex receives more than 90 percent of the total renal blood flow. The paucity of medullary blood flow (its adaptive value for urine concentration will be discussed later) is due to the resistance offered by the vasa recta, but it is not yet possible to quantitate the contributions of the multiple factors (vessel length, blood viscosity, neural tone, chemical mediators, etc.) which cause the resistance in the vasa recta to be higher than in the other intrarenal vessels.

Even more difficult to analyze is the relative distribution of blood flow within the cortex between the juxtamedullary, midcortical, and superficial cortical nephrons. It does seem clear that differences exist and may be subject to physiological control. (The possible significance of this phenomenon for the renal handling of sodium and water is discussed in Chap. 7.) The controlling factors have not been clearly determined, but differences in sympathetic outflow to the arterioles of the various areas of the cortex, as well as differences in autoregulatory responses and prostaglandin-synthesis capabilities of these areas all may be involved.

Study questions: 28 to 33

CHAPTER 6

BASIC RENAL PROCESSES FOR SODIUM, CHLORIDE, AND WATER

OBJECTIVES

The student understands the basic renal processes for sodium, chloride, and water.

1 Calculates or lists the quantities of sodium, chloride, and water normally filtered, reabsorbed, and excreted per day

2 Describes the nature (active or passive) of the process for each substance and the interrelationships between them, i.e., the forces involved; defines transtubular PD and gives its orientation in the different nephron segments

3 Describes the pathway followed by the transported fluid; defines tight junctions and intercellular spaces; states how increased interstitial hydraulic pressure can lead to "back-leakage" in the proximal tubule

4 States the differences in ion transport between the early and the mid-to-late portions of the proximal tubule

5 Describes the mechanism of action of osmotic diuretics; distinguishes osmotic diuresis from water diuresis

6 States the fluid osmolarity and relative water permeability in each nephron segment during water diuresis and antidiuresis

7 Lists the percentages of sodium and water reabsorbed by each nephron segment during antidiuresis and water diuresis

8 Describes the countercurrent multiplier system for urine concentration; states the transport and permeability characteristics of the ascending and descending limbs, the distal tubules and the collecting ducts

9 States the net loss or gain of solute and water for the two limbs of the loop and the collecting duct; states the action of ADH and the nephron sites on which it acts; describes the interaction of ADH and prostaglandins

10 Describes how urea diffusion out of the inner medullary collecting ducts contributes to urine concentrating ability

11 Describes the medullary circulation and its functioning as a countercurrent exchanger

12 States how changes in medullary blood flow or loop flow rates may impede concentration of the urine

13 Describes the obligatory relationships between sodium and water excretion; states how the nephron segments differ in their ability to develop transtubular sodium gradients

Table 1-1 was a typical balance sheet for water; Table 6-1 is the same for sodium. The excretion of sodium via the skin and gastrointestinal tract is normally quite small but may increase markedly during severe sweating, burns, vomiting, diarrhea, or hemorrhage.

Control of the renal excretion of sodium and water constitutes the most important mechanism for the regulation of body sodium and water. The excretory rates of these substances can be varied over an extremely wide range. For example, a consumer of gross amounts of salt may ingest 20 to 25 g of sodium chloride per day, whereas a patient on a low-salt diet may ingest only 50 mg. The normal kidney can readily alter its excretion of salt over this range. Similarly, urinary water excretion can be varied physiologically from approximately 400 mL/day to 25 L/day depending upon whether one is lost in the desert or participating in a beer-drinking contest.

Sodium, chloride, and water are all freely filterable at the glomerulus and undergo considerable tubular reabsorption—normally, more than 99 percent (see Table 2-3)—but no tubular secretion. Most renal energy

Table 6-1 Normal Routes
of Sodium Chloride
Intake and Loss

Route	g/day
Intake	
Food	10.5
Output	
Sweat	0.25
Feces	0.25
Urine	10.0
Total output	10.5

Table 6-2 Summary of Mechanisms By Which Reabsorption of Sodium Drives Reabsorption of Other Substances

---

Reabsorption of sodium:
1. Creates lumen-negative transtubular potential difference that favors reabsorption of anions (e.g., chloride) by diffusion
2. Creates transtubular osmolarity difference which favors reabsorption of water by osmosis; in turn water reabsorption concentrates many luminal solutes (e.g., chloride and urea), thereby favoring their reabsorption by diffusion
3. Achieves reabsorption of many organic nutrients, phosphate, and chloride by co-transport
4. Achieves secretion of hydrogen ion (in the proximal tubule) by countertransport; these hydrogen ions are required for reabsorption of bicarbonate (as described in Chap. 9)

---

utilization goes to accomplish this enormous reabsorptive task. The major tubular mechanisms for reabsorption of these substances can be summarized by three generalizations: (1) The reabsorption of sodium is a primary active process dependent upon the Na-K-dependent ATPase "pumps" in the basolateral membrane. (2) The reabsorption of chloride may be passive and/or active, depending upon the nephron segment, but in either case it is coupled to active reabsorption of sodium. (3) The reabsorption of water is passive (osmosis) and depends upon solute reabsorption, mainly that of sodium. Thus, primary active tubular sodium reabsorption is the primary force that results in reabsorption of chloride and water as well.

SODIUM REABSORPTION AND SODIUM-WATER COUPLING

We described in Chap. 2 the basic pathway for sodium reabsorption; let us do so again, this time emphasizing how the passive reabsorption of water is coupled to it. The key fact to keep in mind is that sodium reabsorption creates the osmotic gradient between lumen and interstitial fluid required to produce net diffusion of water in the same direction.

Recall that luminal sodium ions enter the cell by facilitated diffusion along their electrochemical gradient (Fig. 2-7); the inside of the cell is negatively charged with respect to the lumen, and the intracellular sodium concentration is low because of the active transport of sodium, by the Na-K-dependent ATPase, across the basolateral membrane into the interstitial fluid. Depending upon the nephron segment (Fig. 6-1), sodium's "downhill" movement from lumen into cell may be solely as sodium ions, as co-transport with other substances (glucose, amino acids, chloride, etc.), or as countertransport with other substances (notably hydrogen ion), but the "uphill" step from cell to interstitial fluid is always via the Na-K-dependent ATPase pumps.

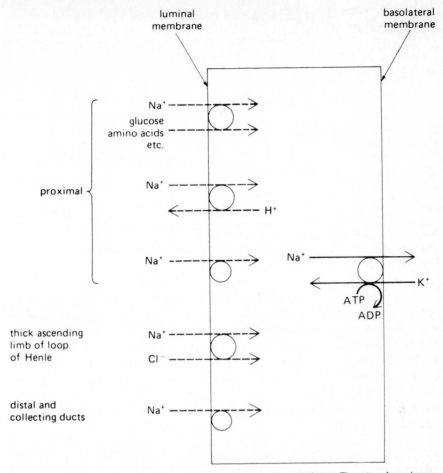

Figure 6-1 Mechanisms of sodium reabsorption along the nephron. The step from lumen to cell is by facilitated diffusion, is always "downhill," and, depending upon the nephron segment, may occur solely as sodium ions or as co- or countertransport with other substances. The "uphill" step across the basolateral membrane is via Na-K-dependent ATPase "pumping" in all nephron segments. At the left, only the most common types of entry are shown for different nephron segments, and this categorization is not meant to be complete.

The movement of sodium from lumen to interstitial fluid lowers total luminal osmolarity (i.e., raises water concentration) and simultaneously raises the osmolarity (lowers the water concentration) in the interstitial fluid. This osmotic gradient from lumen to intercellular space causes net diffusion of water from the lumen across the cell membranes and/or tight junctions into the interstitial fluid (Fig. 6-2).

Table 6-3 Estimated Forces Involved in Movement of Fluid from Interstitium into Capillaries*

Forces	mmHg
1 Favoring uptake	
a Interstitial hydraulic pressure, P_{Int}	3
b Oncotic pressure in peritubular capillaries, π_{PC}	33
2 Opposing uptake	
a Hydraulic pressure in peritubular capillaries, P_{PC}	15
b Interstitial oncotic pressure, π_{Int}	6
3 Net pressure for uptake (1 − 2)	15

*The values for peritubular-capillary hydraulic and oncotic pressures are for the early portions of the capillary. The oncotic pressure, of course, decreases as protein-free fluid enters it, i.e., as absorption occurs, but would not go below 25 mmHg (the value of arterial plasma) even if all fluid originally filtered at the glomerulus were absorbed.

Just how much net osmosis will occur under any given lumen-to-interstitium osmotic gradient is determined by the permeability to water of the cell membranes and tight junctions. The proximal tubule, for example, is so permeable to water that very small gradients suffice to move large quantities of water. In contrast, the distal convoluted tubule is so impermeable to water that almost no water reabsorption occurs no matter how large the osmotic gradient. Finally, and perhaps most important, the water permeability of nephron segments beyond the distal convoluted tubule is not fixed but is subject to physiological control.

To reiterate, water reabsorption is due to differences in osmolarity between lumen and interstitial fluid created by reabsorption of solute.[1] We have dealt only with sodium reabsorption, but the reabsorption of other solutes also contributes to differences in osmolarity and, hence, water reabsorption. However, the reabsorption of most of these other solutes is, itself, ultimately ascribable to sodium reabsorption (Table 6-2). In Chap. 4 we saw that this is true for the many organic substances actively reabsorbed proximally by co-transport with sodium. We shall see, in subsequent sections, that it is also true for almost all chloride reabsorption and most of bicarbonate reabsorption; these are, quantitatively, the only important inorganic anions.

---

[1] To be more accurate, one should refer not just to differences in *absolute* osmolarity, but to differences in *effective* osmolarity. Because of differences in the reflection coefficients of different solutes, it is quite possible to have transtubular differences in effective osmolarity in the absence of differences in absolute osmolarity. For a discussion of this complexity with regard to chloride and bicarbonate see Suggested Readings for Chap. 6.

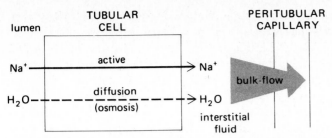

Figure 6-2 Coupling of water and sodium reabsorption. Reabsorption of sodium creates a difference in osmolarity between lumen and interstitial fluid, which causes the diffusion (osmosis) of water in the same direction. The water moves both through and between cells (the latter via the tight junctions). Movement of both solute and water from interstitial fluid into peritubular capillaries occurs by bulk flow.

Thus far we have been describing the movements of sodium and water out of the lumen and into the interstitial fluid. What causes this reabsorbed fluid to move from interstitial fluid into peritubular capillaries (Fig. 6-2)? It is, simply, bulk flow, due to the net balance of hydraulic and oncotic pressures acting across the peritubular capillaries (Table 6-3).

Net pressure for fluid movement into peritubular capillaries is

$$P_{net} = P_{Int} + \pi_{PC} - P_{PC} - \pi_{Int}$$

where the subscripts Int and PC stand for interstitium and peritubular capillary, respectively. This is the second time we have dealt with capillary dynamics in the kidney, the first being the discussion of glomerular filtration. It must be emphasized that the concepts are identical, but, of course, the locations are different. Glomerular dynamics involves the balance of forces between the glomerular capillaries and Bowman's capsule, whereas the peritubular forces are between the interstitium and the peritubular capillaries (Table 6-3). Whereas the net driving pressure across the glomeruli always favors filtration out of the capillaries into Bowman's capsule, the net driving pressure across the peritubular capillaries always favors net movement into the capillaries (reabsorption). The major reason for the latter fact is twofold: (1) The peritubular-capillary hydraulic pressure is generally quite low (10 to 15 mmHg) because the blood entering the peritubular capillaries has already had to flow through the afferent arterioles, glomeruli, and efferent arterioles. (2) The oncotic pressure of the plasma entering the peritubular capillaries is higher than that of the plasma entering the glomeruli because the plasma proteins are concentrated by loss of protein-free filtrate during passage through the glomerular capillaries. (Early peritubular-capillary oncotic pressure is, therefore, identical to end-glomerular-capillary oncotic pressure.)

To reiterate, the final step in fluid reabsorption is bulk flow from interstitium (intercellular spaces) into peritubular capillaries. One of the factors favoring this movement is, as we have seen (Table 6-3), the hydraulic pressure in the interstitial fluid. A crucial new fact is that this hydraulic pressure may, at the same time, produce some "backward" movement of reabsorbed fluid, i.e., bulk flow of interstitial fluid through the tight junctions between cells and back into the lumen. Such back-leakage, of course, reduces the *net* reabsorption of sodium and water, a point to which we shall return in the next chapter.

SODIUM-CHLORIDE COUPLING

How is the *passive* reabsorption of chloride coupled to the active transport of sodium? There are at least two mechanisms responsible for this coupling (Table 6-3). The first mechanism is precisely the same as that previously described for urea. As water moves out of the tubule (secondary to sodium transport), all solutes in the tubule not subject to active transport will increase in concentration. By this means, a chloride transtubular *concentration gradient* is established, which acts as a driving force for chloride reabsorption by diffusion (either simple or facilitated). (You should now recognize that the reabsorption of urea, just as that of chloride, is indirectly coupled to sodium transport via the latter's effect on water reabsorption.)

The second mechanism coupling passive chloride reabsorption to active sodium transport is the *electric potential difference* (PD) that exists across the tubular epithelium. In all nephron segments, with the major exceptions of the ascending thick limb of Henle and the later portions of the proximal tubule, the tubular lumen is negatively charged compared to the interstitial fluid. The magnitude of this lumen-negative PD varies throughout the tubule, ranging from 0 to -4 mV in the early proximal tubule to -40 to -60 mV in portions of the distal tubule. The major contributing factor to this potential is the active reabsorption of sodium. Just on an intuitive level, it should be evident that the active transport of positively charged sodium ions across the epithelium tends to leave the inside of the lumen negatively charged. A systematic analysis of the precise origins of this transtubular PD is beyond the scope of this presentation. What is more important for present purposes is the fact that this PD exists, is contributed to by active sodium transport, and constitutes a driving force for passive chloride reabsorption.

We have, then, both an electric and a chemical (i.e., concentration) difference favoring passive chloride reabsorption. In the proximal tubule, where the PD is very small (and may actually be slightly lumen-positive in its late portions), the concentration difference created by sodium-coupled water transport is most important. In the distal tubules and collecting ducts a very large PD exists and constitutes the major driving force for passive chloride movement.

Thus far we have described only the *passive* reabsorption of chloride. In the thick ascending loop of Henle, chloride reabsorption is a *secondary active process*, and it, too, is coupled to primary active sodium transport (Fig. 6-1). Chloride moves "uphill" across the luminal membrane in co-transport with the simultaneous "downhill" movement of sodium (the latter process supplying the energy for the former), and then out of the cell across the basolateral membrane, probably by simple facilitated diffusion. This is by far the major, perhaps sole, mechanism of chloride reabsorption in the thick ascending loop of Henle. In contrast, a similar process seems also to exist in the late distal tubule and cortical collecting tubules (and possibly other nephron segments as well), but in all these segments it exists side by side with the quantitatively more important passive reabsorptive mechanisms described earlier in this section.

With these generalizations as guides, let us now discuss some of the distinct characteristics of the individual nephron segments relative to salt and water handling.

PROXIMAL TUBULE

The proximal tubule (including both the convoluted and straight portions) is the site of greatest sodium and water reabsorption. Approximately 65 percent of the total filtered sodium and water is reabsorbed by the time the fluid has reached the end of the proximal tubule. Its water permeability is always very great, so passive water reabsorption keeps pace with active sodium reabsorption. The most recent estimate is that only 1 mosmol/L difference between lumen and interstitial fluid can account for most water reabsorption by the proximal tubule. What, therefore, is the concentration of sodium at the end of the proximal tubule? The answer is: almost equal to the plasma sodium concentration. It is true that 65 percent of the mass of sodium filtered has been reabsorbed but so has almost 65 percent of the filtered water. Therefore, the *concentration* of sodium, as opposed to the *mass,* remains virtually unchanged during fluid passage through the proximal tubule.

To reiterate: The proximal reabsorption of sodium is mainly a primary active process, driven by the Na-K-dependent ATPase "pumps" in the basolateral membrane.[2] To illustrate several of the generalizations made

[2] The reason for the word "mainly" in this statement is that in late portions of the proximal tubule, some sodium reabsorption occurs by passive processes — both simple diffusion and solvent drag. I have chosen not to describe this phenomenon because these passive pathways constitute a minor fraction of total proximal sodium reabsorption and because the forces driving them owe their existence ultimately to the usual active sodium transport occurring in earlier proximal segments. (See footnote 3 and Suggested Readings for this chapter.)

earlier, let us look more closely at the interactions between sodium and other solutes along the length of the proximal tubule. In the early portion (Fig. 6-1), a large fraction of the sodium entering the cell across the luminal membrane is via co-transport with organic nutrients (and phosphate). Much of the rest is via countertransport with hydrogen ion; i.e., as sodium ions enter the cell, hydrogen ions are secreted by the same "carrier" into the lumen. As will be described in Chap. 9, these hydrogen ions drive the reabsorption of filtered bicarbonate. Thus, in the early proximal tubule, bicarbonate is the major inorganic anion reabsorbed with sodium, and luminal bicarbonate falls. Simultaneously, water reabsorption is occurring along with solute, but chloride lags behind, so the removal of water causes the luminal chloride concentration to rise substantially. Thus, a transtubular concentration gradient for passive chloride reabsorption is created by the early proximal tubule; accordingly, in the middle and late proximal tubule, chloride is the major anion reabsorbed with sodium.[3]

What is the osmolarity of the fluid at the end of the proximal tubule compared to that of plasma? This is, of course, merely the sum of all the different solute concentrations. Sodium is essentially the same as in plasma, as stressed in preceding paragraphs; chloride is higher and bicarbonate is lower, as described in the previous paragraph; some solutes (like glucose) are lower, whereas others (like urea) are higher. The end result is that the total osmolarity at the end of the proximal tubule is always essentially the same as that of the plasma. This, of course, is not just fortuitous but must be the case, given the extremely high permeability of the proximal tubule to water; i.e., water reabsorption always occurs at a rate that keeps the luminal osmolarity only very slightly less than that of the plasma.

To summarize, during passage through the proximal tubule, approximately 65 percent of the sodium and water are reabsorbed, but the sodium concentration and osmolarity of the fluid remain essentially the same as in plasma. Is there any way to break the tight coupling between sodium and water reabsorption by the proximal tubule? An *osmotic diuretic* is a substance that retards water reabsorption merely because of its osmotic contribution to the tubular fluid. Recall that sodium, chloride, and bicarbonate normally constitute most of the osmotically active solute in plasma. Let us alter the situation by administering to a dog large amounts of the

---

[3] This passive reabsorptive movement of chloride down its electrochemical gradient may be so great in the late proximal tubule that it causes the lumen to become positively charged relative to the interstitium. This lumen-positive potential, in turn, provides a force driving passive reabsorption of sodium. Thus, a fraction of late proximal sodium reabsorption may normally be passive. But note that, if you go back far enough, you will see that this passive reabsorption is traceable to active sodium reabsorption upstream, in the earlier proximal tubule (early proximal sodium reabsorption ➤ early proximal water reabsorption ➤ concentration of luminal chloride ➤ diffusion of chloride out of later proximal tubule ➤ lumen-positive PD ➤ passive sodium reabsorption).

sugar mannitol so that its plasma concentration equals 100 mosmol/L. Mannitol is freely filtered at the glomerulus but is not reabsorbed. In the first portion of the proximal tubule, therefore, mannitol will contribute 100 mosmol/L. As sodium is actively reabsorbed, the total osmolarity of the proximal-tubular fluid begins to decrease, and water, therefore, passively follows the sodium. However, because the mannitol cannot be reabsorbed, its concentration increases as water is reabsorbed. This type of concentrating effect has been previously described for chloride and for urea and obviously will apply to any solute whose reabsorption is slower than that of water. The crucial difference between our experimental conditions and the normal state is that the normally present "lagging" solutes either are present in low concentrations or, like chloride, follow relatively closely behind the water. The mannitol, in contrast, is present in a very large concentration and is not reabsorbed at all. Accordingly, as its concentration rises as a result of water reabsorption, its osmotic presence retards the further reabsorption of water. Thus, passive water movement is prevented from keeping up with active sodium transport. The result is that sodium concentration in the lumen decreases significantly below plasma sodium concentration.

In our discussion of osmotic diuresis we have emphasized the poor reabsorption and increased excretion of water which occurs. Osmotic diuretics also cause the excretion of large quantities of sodium (and chloride), although to a lesser extent than of water. The major reason for this phenomenon illustrates another important characteristic of renal sodium transport: Simultaneously with the *active* transport of sodium out of the tubule, there are occurring quite large fluxes of sodium in both directions by diffusion, since the intercellular junctional complexes are quite permeable to sodium (recall that the proximal tubule is a "leaky" epithelium). But is there a *net diffusional flux* into or out of the proximal tubule? Normally there is very little, since there is no significant transtubular concentration difference for sodium and since the electric potential difference across the proximal tubule is quite small. Therefore, the opposing diffusional fluxes of sodium simply cancel each other out, leaving only the outwardly directed *active* sodium-transport pathway to account for overall *net* sodium movement. However, in the presence of an osmotic diuretic, this situation is altered; because the osmotic diuretic retards water reabsorption, active sodium reabsorption causes the intratubular sodium concentration to decrease as described above. As a result there is a sodium concentration gradient favoring *net* diffusion of sodium from interstitial fluid to lumen. (We are speaking here of sodium *diffusion*, not of the back-leakage by *bulk flow* mentioned earlier.) This net passive influx opposes the active outflux, and so the *overall net* removal of sodium from the proximal-tubular lumen is diminished. This is one of the reasons that osmotic diuretics such as mannitol (or glucose in diabetics) induce the excretion of large quantities of sodium (and chloride) as well as water. The impression should not be left that osmotic diuretics inhibit water and electrolyte reabsorption in the proximal tubule only. In fact, major inhibition also occurs in the loop of Henle (although the mechanism is not exactly the same).

Osmotic diuresis occurs in several diseases, including severe diabetes mellitus. Glucose is normally completely reabsorbed in the proximal tubule. But in patients with uncontrolled diabetes mellitus, the filtered load may exceed the glucose T_m, and large quantities of glucose may remain unreabsorbed. Just like mannitol in the above example, the presence of this glucose retards water and sodium reabsorption and causes an osmotic diuresis.[4] In such a patient, the filtered load of the ketone bodies, acetoacetate and β-hydroxybutyrate, may also exceed the T_ms for these substances so that they also contribute to the osmotic diuresis.

LOOP OF HENLE

The loops of Henle normally reabsorb approximately 25 percent of the filtered sodium and chloride and 15 percent of the filtered water. What percentages of the filtered sodium and water, therefore, enter the distal tubule? The answer is: 10 and 20 percent, respectively, since one must add the quantities reabsorbed by the loop to those already reabsorbed by the proximal tubule to obtain the total quantities unreabsorbed prior to the distal tubule.

As mentioned earlier, the descending limb of Henle (DLH) does not reabsorb sodium or chloride (again the reader is reminded that the terminology used in this book does *not* include the straight portion of the proximal tubule as part of the descending loop of Henle). The entire ascending limb of Henle (ALH), both the thin and thick segments, do reabsorb sodium and chloride. In the thick ALH the reabsorption of sodium is a primary active process involving, as elsewhere, Na-K-dependent ATPase; that of chloride is a secondary active process, the "uphill" step occurring at the luminal membrane as co-transport with "downhill" sodium movement into the cell (Fig. 6-1). Because most sodium movement into the cells of the thick ALH is via this co-transport with chloride, drugs that block this process inhibit the reabsorption not only of chloride but of sodium as well in this nephron segment. The mechanisms of sodium and chloride reabsorption by the thin ALH, in contrast to the thick ALH, are still unclear, as will be discussed below.

---

[4] Recently, it has been demonstrated that hyperglycemia can cause increased urinary excretion of salt and water by mechanisms other than that of classical osmotic diuresis. See Suggested Readings for Chap. 6.

The specific interactions among sodium, chloride, and water in the loop of Henle are complex, and we shall return to them in a subsequent section, since they are so tied up with events in more distal segments. For the moment, it is sufficient to emphasize that the loop, unlike the proximal tubule, *reabsorbs considerably more solute than water.*

DISTAL TUBULE AND COLLECTING DUCT

Recall from Chap. 2 that the terminology for the "distal tubule" is somewhat confusing. Traditionally, renal physiologists have referred to the "distal tubule" as everything between the macula densa and the first junction of two tubules. There is still some merit in retaining this convention because so much micropuncture data is based on it. In doing so, keep in mind that "early distal tubule" refers to the distal convoluted tubule, whereas "late distal tubule" refers to the initial collecting tubule, which has the same structural and functional characteristics as the cortical collecting tubules. Between the distal convoluted tubule and the initial collecting tubule is the connecting segment; except in a few cases, we will not deal specifically with the functional characteristics of this segment, which are generally transitional between the segments on either side of it. One more qualification: The collecting duct system, too, is not homogeneous with respect to its ion-transport characteristics (see Suggested Readings for Chap. 6). However, for the sake of simplicity, in general we shall not deal with these ion-transport differences in this book.

Sodium and chloride reabsorption continues along the distal tubules and collecting ducts so that the final urine normally contains less than 1 percent of the total filtered sodium and chloride. More important than this vague single value—less than 1 percent—is the fact that the exact number is homeostatically regulated (largely by the hormone, aldosterone), depending upon the individual's salt balance, as we shall see in the next chapter. Chloride reabsorption is mainly passive, down its electrochemical gradient (in much of the distal tubule and cortical collecting tubule there is a large transtubular potential, oriented lumen-negative), but there is also a component of active transport (probably co-transport with sodium). This active transport is important for reabsorbing the last bit of chloride from the tubular fluid in states of bodily chloride deficiency.

What about reabsorption of water? The water permeability of the early distal tubule (that portion corresponding to the distal convoluted tubule) is extremely low and unchanging. Accordingly, almost no water is reabsorbed during passage of fluid through it. In contrast, the water permeability of the late distal tubules and the collecting ducts is subject to physiological control (see below) and may vary from extremely low to fairly high (although never as high as that of the proximal tubule).

Let us now combine this information on salt reabsorption and water permeability in following the changes in luminal sodium concentration and osmolarity along the distal tubule and collecting ducts. First, recall that, because more solute than water was reabsorbed in the loop, both the sodium concentration and osmolarity of the fluid entering the distal tubule are well below those of plasma. (The discrepancy is less for osmolarity than for sodium because, as described in Chap. 4, another major solute— urea—is added in the loop.) As fluid flows through the early distal tubule, sodium chloride reabsorption proceeds, but virtually no water is reabsorbed, despite the large osmotic gradient, because of the epithelium's low water permeability. The result is some further lowering of the osmolarity.

Beyond the early distal tubule, i.e., in the late distal tubule and the collecting duct system, the way in which osmolarity changes as the fluid flows along the tubule depends mainly upon the water permeability of the tubule. If the water permeability is very great, so much water is reabsorbed from the late distal tubules and cortical collecting tubules that the luminal fluid once more equilibrates with the plasma in the peritubular capillaries surrounding these structures, i.e., becomes isoosmotic (300 mosmol/L). After equilibrium has occurred, these segments behave analogously to the proximal tubule, reabsorbing approximately equivalent amounts of solute and water. In contrast, when water permeability is low, the hypoosmotic fluid entering the late distal tubule may become even more hypoosmotic as it flows along the tubule, and sodium reabsorption continues, unaccompanied by equivalent water reabsorption.

The water permeability of the medullary collecting ducts shows the same variability as that of the cortical collecting tubules. Thus, in the presence of low permeability, the highly dilute fluid delivered from the cortical collecting tubules remains dilute as it flows through the medullary collecting ducts. In contrast, when the water permeability of the collecting ducts is very great, the isoosmotic fluid leaving the cortical collecting tubules is progressively concentrated in its passage through the medullary collecting ducts. This should come as a surprise since, on the basis of what has been so far described, one ought to conclude that the fluid would merely remain isoosmotic. The explanation will be given in the next section.

The major determinant of water permeability in the late distal tubules and the entire cortical and medullary collecting-duct system is the hormone known as vasopressin, or antidiuretic hormone (ADH). The first name, vasopressin, denotes the fact that, when present in high concentrations, this hormone constricts arterioles and, thereby, increases the arterial blood pressure. The second name describes the effect of the hormone's major renal action—antidiuresis (i.e., against a high urine volume). In the absence of ADH the tubular water permeability is very low, but sodium reabsorption continues, because ADH (at least in physiological concentrations) has relatively little effect on sodium reabsorption[5]; thus, water is unable to follow and remains in the tubule to be excreted as a large volume of urine. On the other hand, in the presence of maximum amounts of ADH, the tubular water permeability is very great, and the final urine volume is small — less than 1 percent of the total filtered water. Of course, the tubular response to ADH is not all-or-none but shows graded increases as the plasma concentration of ADH is increased over a certain range, thus permitting fine adjustments of water permeability and excretion.

The membrane whose water permeability is increased in response to ADH is the luminal membrane, which is rate-limiting for water movement across the entire cell, since its water permeability is so much lower than that of the basolateral membrane. (Why the luminal membrane, in contrast to almost all other plasma membranes, has such a low water permeability in the absence of ADH is not known.) The receptors for ADH are in the basolateral membrane and the binding of ADH by its receptors results in the activation of adenylate cyclase, which catalyzes the intracellular production of cyclic AMP. The sequence of events by which this second messenger then induces increased water permeability of the luminal membrane is not fully understood but most likely involves an increase in the number of membrane protein "channels" through which water can diffuse. Consistent with this concept is the observation (in freeze-fracture studies) that ADH causes the appearance of aggregates of particles in the luminal membrane, perhaps representing a rearrangement of proteins to form water-filled channels.

Interestingly, ADH indirectly exerts a local negative-feedback influence over its own effect. It induces the intramedullary synthesis and release of prostaglandins, which then oppose the action of ADH by interfering with ADH-induced generation of cyclic AMP. Accordingly, abnormal prostaglandin synthesis (either too much or too little) may account for the altered tubular responsiveness to ADH seen in certain renal diseases or during therapy with drugs that block prostaglandin synthesis.[6]

It should now be easy to understand how the kidneys produce a final urine having a lower osmolarity than plasma (hypoosmotic urine), the latter occurring whenever water reabsorption lags behind solute reabsorption, i.e., when plasma ADH is reduced (this is known as *water diuresis*). In this regard, it is worth reemphasizing that, even when virtually no water reabsorption occurs beyond the loop of Henle because of an absence of

[5] For a description of the effects of ADH on electrolyte transport and renal blood flow, see Chap. 5 and Suggested Readings.

[6] Factors other than prostaglandins also influence cell responsiveness to ADH. For example, adrenal steroids also interfere in a variety of ways with ADH's action; therefore, patients with adrenal insufficiency manifest a tendency toward hyperresponsiveness to ADH. This partially explains why such patients reabsorb water excessively, but there are other ADH-independent mechanisms as well (see Suggested Readings for this chapter).

ADH, the reabsorption of sodium is not retarded to any great extent; therefore, intraluminal sodium concentration can be lowered almost to zero in these nephron segments. Recall that the proximal tubule behaves very differently from this when its water reabsorption is blocked, in this case by the presence of an osmotic diuretic; under such conditions net sodium reabsorption is also greatly reduced because of the passive back-leak of sodium from interstitium to lumen. This does not occur to any great extent in the distal tubule and collecting duct because these segments are so much less permeable to sodium; i.e., passive (diffusional) fluxes are very low compared to the rate of active reabsorption. Accordingly, in comparison with the "leaky" proximal tubule, extremely large transtubular gradients for sodium can be achieved by active reabsorption in these "tight" distal segments.

From what has been said so far, one might logically (but wrongly) conclude that it is not possible for the kidneys to produce a hyperosmotic urine, i.e., a urine having an osmolarity greater than that of plasma. For this to occur, is it not necessary for water reabsorption to "get ahead" of solute reabsorption? How can this happen if water reabsorption is always secondary to reabsorption of solute, particularly salt? Yet, as we have mentioned, the kidneys can indeed produce a hyperosmotic urine. Indeed, the final urine may be as concentrated as 1400 mosmol/L compared with a plasma osmolarity of 300 mosmol/L (plasma osmolarity is actually 280 to 290 mosmol/L, but we shall use 300 in this book for ease of calculations). Moreover, this concentrated urine is produced without violating the generalization that water reabsorption is always passive.

URINE CONCENTRATION: THE MEDULLARY COUNTERCURRENT SYSTEM

The ability of the kidneys to produce concentrated urine is not merely an academic problem. It is a major determinant of one's ability to survive without water. The human kidney can produce a maximal urinary concentration of 1400 mosmol/L. The urea, sulfate, phosphate, and other waste products (plus the small number of nonwaste ions) that must be excreted each day amount to approximately 600 mosmol. Therefore, the water required for their excretion constitutes an obligatory water loss and equals:

$$\frac{600 \text{ mosmol/day}}{1400 \text{ mosmol/L}} = 0.429 \text{ L/day}$$

As long as the kidneys are functioning, excretion of this volume of urine will occur, despite the absence of water intake. In a sense, a person lacking access to water may literally urinate to death due to fluid depletion.

If we could produce a urine with an osmolarity of 6000 mosmol/L, then only 100 mL of water need be lost obligatorily each day, and survival time would be greatly expanded. A desert rodent, the kangaroo rat, does just that. This animal never even drinks water because the water produced by oxidation is ample for its needs.

Countercurrent Multiplication

The kidneys produce concentrated urine by a complex interaction of events involving the collecting ducts and the so-called countercurrent multiplier system residing in the loop of Henle. Let us look first at events in the loop and then integrate them with those in the collecting ducts. Recall that the loop of Henle, which is interposed between the proximal and distal tubules, is a hairpin loop extending into the renal medulla. Let us list the critical characteristics of this loop:

1 As described in Chap. 1, the ascending limb of the loop (i.e., the limb leading to the distal tubule) is not a structurally homogenous segment. It is very thin from the bend in the loop up to the outer medulla (only long loops have this thin ascending portion), where it becomes much thicker. This structural difference reflects functional differences as well. However, for simplicity, we initially present the physiological characteristics of the thick portion as though they apply to the entire ascending limb; afterwards, the necessary qualification will be made. As stated earlier in this chapter the thick ascending limb actively transports sodium and chloride out of the tubular lumen into the surrounding interstitium; i.e., it reabsorbs these ions. However, the ascending limb is always quite impermeable to water so that water cannot follow the sodium chloride.

2 The descending limb of the loop (i.e., the limb into which drains fluid from the proximal tubule) does *not actively* transport either chloride or sodium. Moreover, it has a very great permeability to water but is relatively impermeable to the ions.

Keeping these characteristics in mind, and assuming that the entire ascending limb has the characteristics of the thick segment, imagine the loop of Henle filled with a stationary column of fluid supplied by the proximal tubule. At first, the concentration everywhere would be 300 mosmol/L, since fluid leaving the proximal tubule is isoosmotic to plasma.

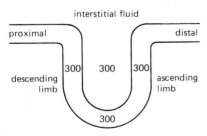

Now let the active pump in the ascending limb transport sodium chloride into the interstitium until a limiting gradient (say, 200 mosmol/L) is established between ascending-limb fluid and interstitium.

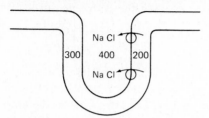

A limiting gradient is reached because the ascending limb is relatively permeable to sodium and chloride. Accordingly, passive back flux into the lumen counterbalances active outflux, and a steady-state limiting gradient is established.

Given the great permeability of the descending limb to water, there is a net diffusion of water[7] out of the descending limb and into the interstitium until the osmolarities are equal. The interstitial osmolarity is maintained at 400 mosmol/L during this equilibration because of continued sodium chloride transport out of the ascending limb.

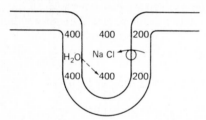

Note that the osmolarities of the descending limb and interstitium are equal and both are higher than that of the ascending limb. So far we have held the fluid stationary in the loop, but, of course, it is actually continuously flowing. Let us look at what occurs under conditions of flow (Fig. 6-3). We shall simplify the analysis by assuming that flow through the loop, on the one hand, and ion and water movements, on the other, occur in discontinuous, out-of-phase steps. During the stationary phase, as described above, sodium chloride is transported out of the ascending limb to establish a gradient of 200 mosmol/L, and water diffuses out of the descending limb until descending limb and interstitium have the same osmolarity. During the flow phase, fluid leaves the loop via the distal tubule, and new fluid enters the loop from the proximal tubule.

---

[7] The descending limb is not completely impermeable to sodium and chloride. Accordingly, some of these ions diffuse into the loop simultaneously with water movement out of the loop. For simplicity, we ignore this additional complexity. (See Kokko, 1974, in Suggested Readings for Chap. 6.)

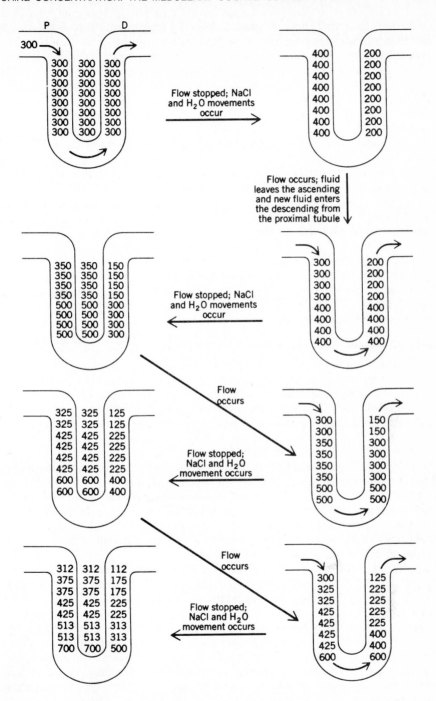

Figure 6-3 Countercurrent multiplier system in loop of Henle. *(Redrawn from R. F. Pitts, Physiology of the Kidney and Body Fluids, 3d ed., Year Book, Chicago, 1974.)*

Note that the fluid is progressively concentrated as it flows down the descending limb and then is progressively diluted as it flows up the ascending limb. While a gradient of only 200 mosmol/L is maintained across the ascending limb at any given *horizontal level* in the medulla, there exists a much larger osmotic gradient from the top of the medulla to the bottom (312 mosmol/L versus 700 mosmol/L). In other words, the gradient of 200 mosmol/L established by active ion transport has been *multiplied* because of the *countercurrent* flow (i.e., flow in opposing directions through the two limbs of a loop) within the loop. It should be emphasized that the active-ion-transport mechanism within the ascending limb is the essential component of the entire system; without it, the countercurrent flow would have no effect whatsoever on concentrations.

The highest concentration achieved at the tip of the loop depends upon many factors, particularly the length of the loop (the kangaroo rat has extremely long loops) and the strength of the ion pump. In humans, the value reached is 1400 mosmol/L, which, you will recall, is also the maximal concentration of the excreted urine. But what has this system really accomplished? Certainly, it concentrates the loop fluid to 1400 mosmol/L, but then it immediately redilutes the fluid so that the fluid entering the distal tubule is actually more dilute than the plasma. Where is the *final urine* concentrated and how?

The site of final concentration is in the medullary collecting ducts. Recall that the collecting ducts course through the renal medulla, parallel to the loops of Henle, and are bathed by the interstitial fluid of the medulla. As described above, in the presence of maximal levels of ADH, fluid leaves the cortical collecting tubules isoosmotic to plasma, i.e., at 300 mosmol/L. As this fluid flows through the medullary collecting ducts, it equilibrates with the everincreasing osmolarity of the interstitial fluid. Thus, the real function of the loop countercurrent multiplier system is to concentrate the *medullary interstitium*. Under the influence of ADH, the collecting ducts are highly permeable to water, which diffuses out of the collecting ducts and into the interstitium as a result of the osmotic gradient (Fig. 6-4). The net result is that the fluid at the end of the collecting duct has equilibrated with the interstitial fluid at the tip of the medulla. In contrast, in the presence of low plasma-ADH concentrations, the collecting ducts become relatively impermeable to water, and the interstitial osmotic gradient is ineffective in inducing water movement out of them.

Because the osmolarity of the urine becomes greater than that of plasma only in the medullary collecting ducts, it is easy to forget that ADH acts not only on this segment but on the late distal tubules and cortical collecting tubules as well. The action on these segments is equally important because by permitting the reabsorption there of a relatively large quantity of fluid, it ensures the delivery to the medullary collecting ducts of a volume of isoosmotic fluid small enough for efficient concentrating.

Let us summarize the overall net movement of sodium chloride and water out of the tubules and into the medullary interstitium during formation of a concentrated urine. First, sodium chloride is lost from the ascending

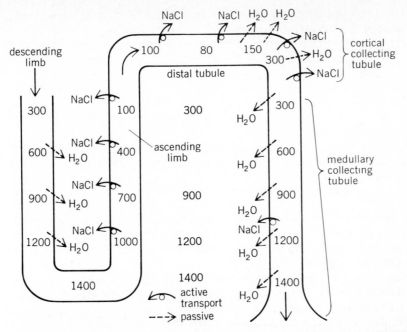

Figure 6-4 Interactions of loop of Henle and collecting duct in formation of a concentrated urine. Note that interstitial osmolarity at every level is identical to descending-limb and collecting-duct osmolarity. As described in the text, this figure is oversimplified in that it assumes active transport by the entire ascending loop and ignores the role of urea.

limb by active transport of sodium[8] and chloride. This sodium chloride causes net diffusion of water out of the descending limb and the collecting ducts. In the steady state, this sodium chloride and water entering the medullary interstitium must be taken up by capillaries and carried away. This is, of course, the final step during reabsorption of fluid anywhere in the tubules, and it occurs as a result of the usual hydraulic and oncotic forces acting across the capillary wall.

As noted, the above description of the countercurrent multiplier system ignored the fact that the thin ascending loop of Henle may function differently from the thick ascending loop, specifically that it probably does not actively reabsorb sodium and chloride (the evidence for or against this is presently not decisive). Should this prove to be the case, what is the mechanism by which sodium chloride leaves the thin ascending limb? (That sodium chloride *does* move from the lumen of the thin ascending limb into the interstitium is well established—the question at hand here deals only with what the force is that causes these ions to move.) Several hypotheses

---

[8] As described earlier, sodium is also actively reabsorbed from the collecting ducts. This phenomenon helps to reduce the amount of salt lost to the urine. But it has been ignored in our analysis because it is not an important component of the countercurrent system. (See Giebisch and Windhager, 1973, in Suggested Readings for Chap. 6.)

Table 6-4 Composition of Medullary Interstitial Fluid and Urine During Formation of a Concentrated Urine

Interstitial fluid at tip of medulla (mosmol/L)	Urine (mosmol/L)
Urea = 650 $Na^+ + Cl^- = 750^*$	Urea = 700 Non-urea solutes = 700 (Na^+, Cl^-, K^+, urate, creatinine, etc.)

*Some other ions (e.g., potassium) contribute, to a small degree, to this osmolarity.

other than active transport have been postulated, but none of them alone can presently explain all the data; they generally invoke a special role for urea, and the interested reader should consult the articles cited in the Suggested Readings for this chapter.

Regardless of whether urea is somehow involved in the movement of sodium chloride out of the ascending thin limb, it is definitely involved in another way in the urine-concentrating mechanism, specifically in determining the maximal osmolarity of the urine. From the description of the counter-current multiplier system given thus far, one would logically assume that all the solutes in the medullary interstitial fluid are sodium and chloride. Such is not the case, for approximately half of the medullary osmolarity consists of urea. However, this should not really be surprising when you recall from Chap. 4 how urea is handled beyond the loop of Henle. Luminal urea concentration rises progressively along the distal tubules, cortical collecting tubules, and the outer medullary collecting tubules (as water is reabsorbed but urea is not because these tubular segments are impermeable to it). This high urea concentration then drives diffusion out of the inner medullary collecting tubules, which are highly permeable to urea. (The simultaneous movement of water out of the inner medullary collecting tubules maintains a high urea concentration even as urea is being lost from the tubule.) The net result is that the urea concentration of the inner medullary interstitial fluid comes to approximate the urea concentration of the luminal fluid within adjacent medullary collecting tubules. In essence, then, urea within the tubule is balanced by urea within the interstitium; therefore, the sodium and chloride within the interstitium need balance only the solutes other than urea in the tubular fluid. Thus, typical values for the case in which a highly concentrated urine is being formed are shown in Table 6-4. Note that if there were no urea in the interstitial fluid, then the interstitial osmolarity due to sodium and chloride would have to be 1400, rather than 750; i.e., more sodium chloride would have to be transported by the ascending loop of Henle.

In this description, it is easy to lose track of an essential point: Urea, unlike the sodium and chloride reabsorbed out of the ascending loop of

Henle, does not cause water to move from tubular lumen to medullary interstitium. It balances itself but does not cause concentration of any other solute.

Countercurrent Exchange: Vasa Recta

There is a unique characteristic of the medullary circulation without which the entire system could not operate, namely, the hairpin-loop anatomy of certain of the medullary vessels, of the *vasa recta*, which run parallel to the loops of Henle and medullary collecting ducts (Fig. 6-5). The problem is this: What would happen to the medullary gradient if the medulla were supplied only with ordinary capillaries? As plasma having the usual osmolarity of 300 mosmol/L entered the highly concentrated environment of the medulla, there would be massive net diffusion of sodium chloride into the capillaries and of water out of them. Thus, the interstitial gradient would soon be lost. But, with hairpin loops, the sequence of events shown in Fig. 6-5 occurs. Blood enters the vessel loop at an osmolarity of 300 mosmol/L, and as it flows down the capillary loop deeper and deeper into the medulla, sodium chloride does indeed diffuse into, and water out of, the vessel. However, after the bend in the loop is reached, the blood then flows up the ascending vessel loop, where the process is almost completely reversed. Thus, the vessel loop is acting as a so-called *countercurrent exchanger*, which prevents the gradient from being dissipated. Note that the vessel is, itself, completely passive; i.e., it is not *creating* the medullary gradient, only protecting it. Its passive nature explains why it is called an exchanger; compare its function to that of the loop of Henle, which actively creates the gradient and is, therefore, a multiplier. Finally, it should be noted that the hairpin-loop structure minimizes losses of solute or water from the interstitium by *diffusion*. It does not, though, prevent the *bulk flow* of medullary interstitial fluid into the capillaries secondary to the usual Starling forces. By this bulk-flow process, the net salt and water entering the interstitium from the loops and collecting ducts is carried away, and the steady-state gradient is maintained.

Clinical Changes in Urinary Concentrating Ability

A point of considerable clinical importance is that inability to achieve maximal urinary concentration occurs early in any renal disease because of interference with the establishment of the medullary gradient. Any significant change in renal structure, particulary in the medulla, can upset the intricate geometric relationships required for maximal countercurrent functioning. A change in renal blood flow to the medulla, either too much or too little, will reduce the gradient by carrying away too much or too little water and/or solute. Destruction of the loops will also reduce the gradient, as will decreased sodium and chloride pumping by the ascending limb. The

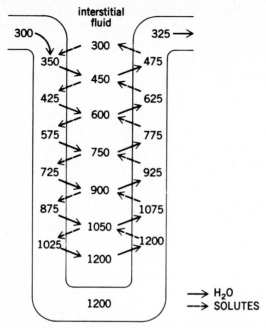

Figure 6-5 Vasa recta as countercurrent exchangers. *(Redrawn from R. F. Pitts, Physiology of the Kidney and Body Fluids, 3d ed., Year Book, Chicago, 1974.)*

latter may be caused by tubular disease or by a marked reduction in GFR and, thereby, a reduction in the supply of sodium and chloride to the loop. Another important factor is flow rate through the loop; any large increase (as, for example, in osmotic diuresis) literally "washes out" the gradient, thereby preventing concentration of the final urine.

Finally, it should be emphasized that, although the entire discussion of renal concentrating ability has been in terms of urine osmolarity, the usual clinical measurement of urine "concentration" is *specific gravity*. The determination of specific gravity requires only a hydrometer and is easy and cheap to perform. However, specific gravity is really a measure of urine density, not of concentration. Frequently, the two correlate well, but under certain circumstances they can be quite divergent, since specific gravity is influenced by the nature as well as by the number of solute particles. For example, protein in the urine causes the specific gravity to be increased with little change in osmolarity.

SUMMARY

Figure 6-6 summarizes the previously described changes in volume and osmolarity of the tubular fluid as it flows along the nephron.

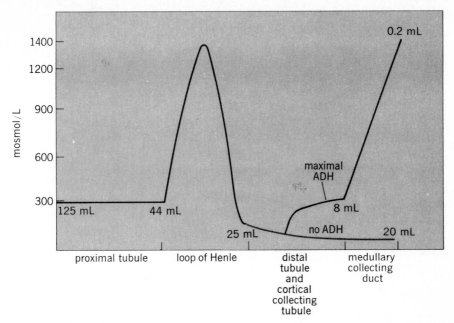

Figure 6-6 Changes in volume and osmolarity of the tubular fluid as it flows along the nephron.

1 Approximately 65 percent of the filtered water and sodium chloride are reabsorbed in the proximal tubule, but the fluid remains isoosmotic.

2 In the loop, water is reabsorbed from the descending limb, but much more sodium chloride is reabsorbed from the ascending limb so that hypoosmotic fluid enters the distal tubule.

3 Fluid remains hypoosmotic in the early distal tubule with little or no water reabsorption occurring. Thus, the ascending loop of Henle and early distal tubule are often referred to as "diluting segments."

4 Only from the late distal tubules on does the presence or absence of ADH matter. With essentially no ADH, very little water is reabsorbed from the late distal tubules and collecting ducts (and these segments therefore also contribute to dilution of the urine). Consequently, a large volume of dilute urine is formed.

5 With maximal ADH, water reabsorption is high in the late distal tubules and collecting ducts. By the end of the cortical portions of the collecting duct system (the cortical collecting tubules), the fluid has once more become isoosmotic. Almost all the remaining water is reabsorbed in the medullary collecting ducts, and a tiny volume of highly concentrated urine is formed. Because of the focus on sodium chloride in this chapter, the reader may be surprised to discover that a maximally concentrated urine (1400 mosmol/L) may, under certain conditions, contain virtually no sodium chloride; the solute may be urea, creatinine, uric acid, potassium, etc. In other words, although sodium chloride *in the medullary interstitium* is the essential requirement for pulling water out of the collecting ducts and concentrating the urine, there need be no sodium chloride in the urine itself.

Several other points of great importance should be reemphasized: (1) Excretion of large quantities of sodium *always* results in the excretion of large quantities of water. This follows from the passive nature of water reabsorption since water can be reabsorbed only if sodium is reabsorbed first. As we shall see, this relationship has considerable importance for the regulation of extracellular volume. (2) In contrast, large quantities of water can be excreted even though the urine is virtually free of sodium since a decreased ADH will increase water excretion without altering sodium transport significantly. This process we shall find crucial for the renal regulation of extracellular osmolarity.

Given the basic renal processes for handling sodium, chloride, and water, we now turn to the mechanisms by which they are controlled so as to homeostatically regulate salt and water balance.

Study Questions: 34 to 43

CONTROL OF SODIUM AND WATER EXCRETION: REGULATION OF EXTRACELLULAR VOLUME AND OSMOLARITY

OBJECTIVES

The student understands the renal regulation of extracellular volume and osmolarity.

1 States the formula relating filtration, reabsorption, and excretion of sodium

2 Describes the nature and locations of receptors in sodium-regulating reflexes

3 Lists the efferent inputs controlling GFR and how these inputs change as a result of changes in sodium balance or fluid volumes

4 Defines glomerulotubular balance and describes its significance

5 States the origin of aldosterone, its sites of action, and its effects

6 Lists the factors controlling aldosterone secretion and states which is most important

7 Defines natriuretic hormone

8 Describes how peritubular-capillary dynamics (physical factors) influence sodium reabsorption; states how changes in filtration fraction influence sodium reabsorption; predicts the changes in physical factors that occur with changes in sodium or fluid balance and how they alter sodium and water reabsorption

9   Defines redistribution of blood flow and states how it might influence sodium and water excretion

10   States all direct and indirect effects of catecholamines and angiotensin II on sodium reabsorption

11   Lists all the actions of angiotensin II that increase arterial blood pressure

12   Distinguishes between primary and secondary hyperaldosteronism; describes the hormonal changes in each and the presence or absence of "escape"

13   Describes the origin of ADH and the reflex controls of its secretion; defines diabetes insipidus; states the effects of ADH on arterioles

14   Distinguishes between the reflex changes that occur when an individual has suffered fluid loss because of diarrhea as opposed to a pure water loss, i.e., solute-water loss as opposed to pure-water loss

15   Calculates the changes in body-fluid volumes and osmolarity resulting from the excretion of a known volume of urine having a given osmolarity; defines and, given data, calculates free-water clearance (both positive and negative)

16   Describes the control of thirst

17   Diagrams in flow-sheet form the pathways by which sodium and water excretion are altered in response to sweating, diarrhea, hemorrhage, high- or low-salt diet

Since sodium is freely filterable at the glomerulus and actively reabsorbed but not secreted by the tubules, the amount of sodium excreted in the final urine represents the results of two processes, glomerular filtration and tubular reabsorption:

$$\text{Sodium excretion} = \text{sodium filtered} - \text{sodium reabsorbed}$$
$$= (\text{GFR} \times P_{\text{Na}}) - \text{sodium reabsorbed}$$

It is possible, therefore, to adjust sodium excretion by controlling any of these three variables (Fig. 7-1).

P_{Na} may change considerably in several pathological conditions, and these changes can influence sodium excretion. However, under most physiological situations, P_{Na} changes very little (except to increase transiently after a sodium-rich meal or decrease transiently after drinking a large quantity of fluid containing no sodium) and may be disregarded as an important control point for regulation of sodium excretion. Accordingly, control is exerted mainly on the other two variables—GFR and sodium reabsorption.

What happens if the quantity of filtered sodium increases as a result of a higher GFR but the rate of reabsorption remains constant? Clearly, sodium excretion increases. The same final result could be achieved by lowering sodium reabsorption while the GFR remains constant. Finally, sodium excretion could be raised greatly by elevating the GFR and simultaneously reducing reabsorption. Conversely, sodium excretion could be decreased below normal levels by lowering the GFR or by raising sodium reabsorption, or by both.

FILTERED   REABSORBED   EXCRETED
Na⁺   Na⁺   Na⁺

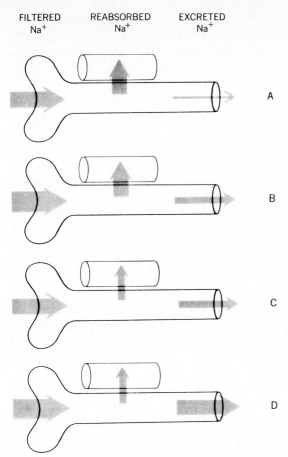

Figure 7-1 Sodium excretion is increased by increasing the GFR (B), by decreasing reabsorption (C), or by a combination of both (D). The arrows indicate relative magnitudes of filtration, reabsorption, and excretion. (*From A. J. Vander et al., Human Physiology,* © *1970 by McGraw-Hill, Inc. Used with permission of McGraw-Hill Book Company.*)

The reflex pathways by which changes in total body sodium balance lead to changes in GFR and sodium reabsorption include: (1) "volume" receptors and the afferent pathways leading from them to the central nervous system and endocrine glands; (2) efferent neural and hormonal pathways to the kidneys; and (3) renal effector sites, i.e., the renal arterioles and tubules.

The first component of the reflexes, the so-called volume receptors, offers certain theoretical difficulties. In most physiological control mechanisms, reflexes regulating the magnitude of any given variable (plasma glucose, Po_2, etc.) are initiated by receptors sensitive to changes in that variable. One might, therefore, have expected that reflexes which regulate sodium balance would involve sodium receptors. As we shall see, there are sodium-sensitive receptors in various locations of the body (notably in the adrenal cortex, macula densa of the renal tubules, and brain), but they are not the most important receptors in sodium-controlling reflexes. However, this should not really be too surprising, since what is being held constant by these reflexes is not the *concentration* of sodium in the body fluids but the *total mass* of sodium in the body. Therefore, one must look for some other variable that correlates closely with total body sodium and that might constitute the critical signal. As shown in the following examples, the ideal candidate is the volume of extracellular fluid.

What happens when a person ingests a liter of isotonic sodium chloride, i.e., a solution of salt with exactly the same osmolarity as the body fluids? It is absorbed from the gastrointestinal tract into the plasma, from which most of it then enters the interstitial fluid. The important fact is that all the salt and water remain in the extracellular fluid (plasma and interstitial fluid) and none enters the cells. Because of the active sodium pumps in cell membranes, sodium is effectively barred from the cells. The water, too, remains extracellular since only the volume and not the osmolarity of the extracellular compartment has been changed; i.e., no osmotic gradient exists to drive the ingested water into cells. Another example: A person ingests 145 mmol of sodium chloride but no water. The salt is distributed in the extracellular fluid but is barred from the cells. The addition of this water-free solute to the extracellular fluid causes extracellular osmolarity to rise above intracellular osmolarity; therefore, water diffuses out of the cells and into the extracellular fluid until the osmolarities are once more equal. The net result is an expansion of extracellular volume and a decrease of intracellular volume.

These examples lead us to the extremely important generalization that the total extracellular-fluid volume depends primarily upon the mass of extracellular sodium, which, in turn, correlates directly with total body sodium, since sodium is effectively barred from cells. (There are considerable amounts of sodium in bone, but this fact does not seriously alter the analysis.) It should now be clear why reflexes that maintain extracellular volume constant simultaneously keep total body sodium constant in normal persons.

Yet how can there be receptors capable of detecting changes in the total extracellular volume? The answer is almost certainly that there are not any and that total extracellular volume per se is not *directly* monitored. What about its component volumes — plasma volume and interstitial volume? Again neither of these is *directly* monitored; instead, the variables monitored in sodium-regulating reflexes are those that are altered as a result of changes in these volumes (Fig. 7-2) — notably *intravascular* and *intracardiac* pressures. For example, a decrease in plasma volume generally tends to lower the hydraulic pressures within the veins, cardiac chambers, and arteries; these changes are detected by baroreceptors within all those structures, and initiate the reflexes leading to renal sodium retention, which helps restore the plasma volume toward normal. As shown in Fig. 7-2, other derivatives of extracellular volume that might be detected are organ blood flows and interstitial pressures; however, a role for these variables and others that have been postulated has not been convincingly documented.

To recapitulate, receptors sensitive to sodium (or chloride) do exist and contribute to the regulation of total body sodium, but the major receptors involved in this regulation are those which respond to changes in pressure (or distention) in the cardiovascular system. In the normal person, regulation of these variables results in excellent homeostasis of body sodium and extracellular-fluid volume, since these parameters are all so dependent upon one another. However, as we shall see, disease states can produce striking discrepancies between them with a resulting abnormal expansion of extracellular volume and total body sodium.

Several qualifications should be added to this general scheme. First, this entire description has been in terms of "reflexes," but the fact is, as we shall see, several of the receptors cited are within the kidneys themselves, and no "reflex" input to or output from the kidneys is required in the sequences of events they elicit. Second, the kidneys are influenced directly by changes in the blood perfusing them—for example, by oncotic pressure—so that such nonreflex inputs related to altered sodium balance are also important in determining sodium excretion.

CONTROL OF GFR

The control of GFR has already been described, first in Chap. 2 (which dealt with the factors directly determining GFR) and Chap. 5 (which dealt with the neuroendocrine regulation of these factors). Accordingly, this section is simply a review of the salient features of those descriptions in the specific context of reflexes regulating sodium and water excretion.

Physiological Regulation of Glomerular-Capillary Pressure

Let us take a specific example: What changes in renal hemodynamics occur as a result of severe salt and water loss due to diarrhea (Fig. 7-3)? The decreased plasma volume resulting from salt and water loss prevents adequate venous return, thereby reducing atrial pressure, cardiac output, and arterial blood pressure. The fall in arterial blood pressure decreases filtration rate by lowering glomerular-capillary hydraulic pressure. Recall, however, that, because of renal autoregulation, arterial-pressure

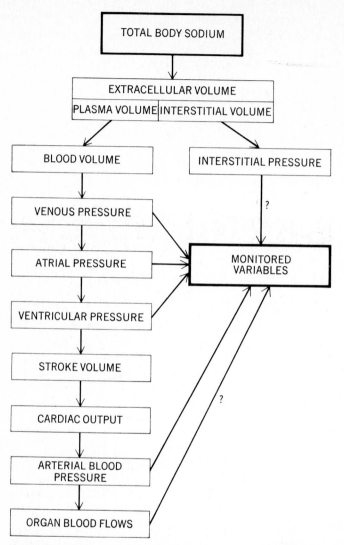

Figure 7-2 Flow sheet demonstrating the series of derivative variables dependent upon total body sodium. In no case is any block in the sequence totally dependent upon the previous one, for other factors are also involved. The major aim of the figure is to demonstrate how a change in body sodium could result in changes in a group of monitored variables that could be detected by receptors and initiate the responses controlling sodium excretion.

changes per se have only small effects on GFR over the usual physiological range.

However, the drops in blood pressure are also detected by the carotid sinuses and aortic arch, as well as by other baroreceptors in the veins

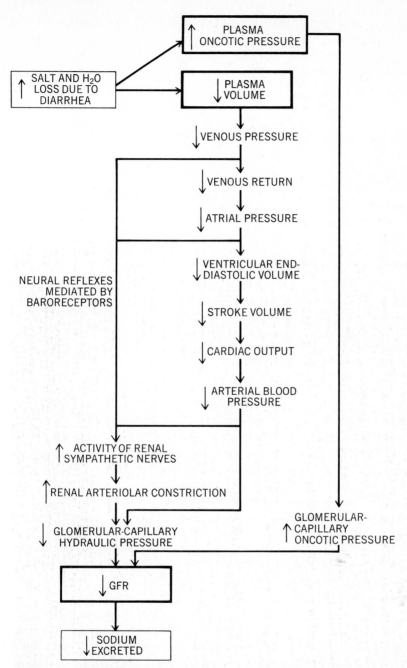

Figure 7-3 Several major pathways by which the GFR is decreased when plasma volume decreases. The baroreceptors that initiate the sympathetic reflex are probably located in large veins and in the walls of the heart, as well as in the carotid sinuses and aortic arch. For clarity, circulating catecholamines and the renin-angiotensin system, both of which lower GFR, have not been included in the figure, nor have the effects of these inputs on glomerular K_f (see text). (*Modified from A. J. Vander et al., Human Physiology, © 1970 by McGraw-Hill, Inc. Used with permission of McGraw-Hill Book Company.*)

and atria. The information (decreased firing rate of the baroreceptors) is relayed to the medullary cardiovascular centers, which respond by inhibiting parasympathetic outflow to the heart and by stimulating sympathetic outflow to the heart and to arteriolar smooth muscle. The sympathetic stimulation of the renal arterioles (both by the renal nerves and by epinephrine from the adrenal medulla) increases constriction of the renal arterioles. The vasoconstriction of the afferent arterioles increases the resistance to blood flow from the renal artery to the glomerular capillaries, lowering the capillary blood pressure and GFR. (As described in Chap. 5, increased sympathetic activity also causes some efferent-arteriolar constriction, which tends to increase glomerular-capillary hydraulic pressure, but the afferent effect usually predominates.)

By this mechanism, both the amount of sodium filtered and the amount of sodium excreted are reduced, and further loss from the body is prevented. Conversely, an increased GFR can result reflexly from greater plasma volume and contribute to increased renal sodium loss, which returns extracellular volume to normal.

In this discussion we have emphasized the significance of the sympathetic nervous system as a major efferent pathway for GFR regulation. As described in Chap. 5, under the conditions of our example, renin secretion would also be stimulated, so that increased plasma angiotensin II would contribute to renal vasoconstriction.

Physiological Changes in Plasma Protein Concentration

There are frequent situations in which changes in plasma or extracellular volume are associated with changes in plasma protein concentration. In such situations, changes in glomerular-capillary oncotic pressure may also play an important role in the physiological raising or lowering of GFR. For example, the severe fluid loss of sweating or diarrhea (Fig. 7-3) will lower the extracellular volume, but at the same time it will concentrate plasma protein. The resulting increase in oncotic pressure will reduce net filtration pressure in the glomeruli and, thereby, GFR. Conversely, a marked increase in salt intake will increase extracellular volume and, at least transiently, lower plasma protein concentration. The result is lowered oncotic pressure and increased GFR.

In each of these examples, the change in arterial-plasma protein concentration is in the appropriate direction to reestablish salt balance by decreasing or increasing salt excretion. Is this also true for hemorrhage? The answer is *no*. Hemorrhage per se does not immediately alter plasma protein concentration, since all blood components are lost in equivalent proportions. However, the blood loss is followed by a net movement of interstitial fluid into the vascular compartment. This entry of protein-free fluid lowers the arterial-plasma protein concentration, which tends to raise GFR — an inappropriate response, since sodium conservation, not increased sodium loss, is the "desired" response to hemorrhage. However, GFR does decrease in response to hemorrhage despite the fact that oncotic pressure is going in the wrong direction. Why? Because decreased arterial pressure and reflexly increased sympathetic outflow to the afferent arterioles cause glomerular-capillary pressure to fall by a larger amount than oncotic pressure falls. This example is presented as a reminder of the fact that the GFR response to any given situation represents the algebraic sum of multiple forces.

Physiological Control of Glomerular Filtration Coefficient (K_f)

In Chap. 2, it was described how, at any given net filtration pressure, GFR is proportional to the glomerular filtration coefficient (K_f). The catecholamines and angiotensin II are known to reduce K_f (either directly or via an intrarenal mediator) by causing mesangial cells to contract, and it is likely that this action contributes to the GFR-lowering effects of these neuroendocrine inputs.

CONTROL OF TUBULAR SODIUM REABSORPTION

Present evidence indicates that, so far as long-term regulation of sodium excretion is concerned, the control of tubular sodium reabsorption is probably more important than that of GFR (even though, as we shall see, the former is somewhat dependent on the latter). For example, patients with chronic marked reductions of GFR usually maintain normal sodium excretion by decreasing tubular sodium reabsorption.

Glomerulotubular Balance

One reason for the lesser importance of changes in the filtered load of sodium is the fact that the absolute reabsorption of fluid in the proximal tubules, and probably the loops of Henle and distal tubules as well, varies directly with glomerular filtration rate. This phenomenon is known as *glomerulotubular balance*. (Recall that one of the likely mechanisms for GFR autoregulation is known as *tubulo-glomerular feedback*, a name unfortunately very easy to confuse with the totally different phenomenon of *glomerulotubular balance* being described here.) For example, if GFR is experimentally decreased by 25 percent (by tightening a clamp around the renal artery), the absolute rate of proximal fluid reabsorption is observed to decrease by almost the same percentage. Another way of saying this is that the percentage of the filtrate reabsorbed proximally remains approximately constant (at 65 percent). The mechanisms responsible for adjusting tubular reabsorption to GFR are not

Table 7-1   Effect of "Perfect" Glomerulotubular Balance on the Mass of Sodium Leaving the Proximal Tubule

GFR, L/min	P_{Na}, mmol/L	Filtered, mmol/min	Reabsorbed proximally (66.7% of filtered), mmol/min	Leaving proximal, mmol/min
0.124	145	18	12	6
0.165	145	24	16	8
0.062	145	9	6	3

clear. (Part of the explanation is simply that when GFR is increased, there is an increased supply of substances co-transported with sodium — glucose, amino acids, etc. — to later portions of the proximal tubule.) It is certain, however, that they are completely intrarenal; i.e., glomerulotubular balance requires no external neural or hormonal input and can be shown to occur in a completely isolated kidney. The net effect of this phenomenon is to *blunt* the ability of GFR changes per se to produce *large* changes in sodium excretion. However, for several reasons, it is incorrect to assume that, because of glomerulotubular balance, sodium excretion is *completely* unaffected by changes in filtered load. First, even if glomerulotubular balance were perfect, i.e., if the changes in GFR and reabsorption were exactly proportional, the *absolute* amounts of sodium leaving the proximal tubule would still change when GFR changes; this can be seen in the example given in Table 7-1 — even though reabsorption stays fixed at 66.7 percent, the amount of sodium leaving the proximal tubule rises when GFR is increased and falls when GFR is decreased. Second, glomerulotubular balance is not really perfect; i.e., the changes in GFR and reabsorption are not usually exactly proportional. The proper conclusion is that changes in the filtered load of sodium per se do result in changes in sodium excretion, but the changes are greatly mitigated by glomerulotubular balance.

In a sense, glomerulotubular balance is a second line of defense preventing changes in hemodynamics per se from causing large changes in sodium excretion. The first line of defense is autoregulation of GFR. In other words, autoregulation prevents GFR from changing too much in direct response to changes in blood pressure, and glomerulotubular balance blunts the sodium-excretion response to whatever GFR change does occur. Glomerulotubular balance allows major responsibility for control of sodium excretion to reside in those factors, to be described next, which act specifically to influence tubular reabsorption of sodium above and beyond any change induced directly by GFR changes. We also see here another analogy between autoregulation and glomerulotubular balance in that both are manifest in their "pure" forms only when the kidneys are manipulated in relative isolation from the rest of the body, as by altering renal perfusion through the use of renal-artery clamps. In contrast, when GFR is made to change by doing something to the whole animal or person, say by infusing large quantities of isotonic saline, glomerulotubular balance can be overridden by other inputs to the kidney so that the proximal tubule is observed to reabsorb a smaller percentage (in our saline-infusion example) or a larger percentage (in situations like severe hemorrhage) than usual.

Aldosterone

A major clue to the single most important controller of sodium reabsorption was the observation that patients whose adrenal glands are diseased or missing excrete large quantities of sodium in the urine. Indeed, if untreated, they may die because of low blood pressure resulting from depletion of plasma volume. This increased sodium excretion often occurs despite lowered GFR, thus establishing that decreased tubular reabsorption is the factor responsible for the sodium loss. The adrenal influence on sodium reabsorption is mediated by a hormone, *aldosterone,* produced by the *adrenal cortex,* specifically in the cortical area known as the *zona glomerulosa.* (This term is somewhat unfortunate because it sounds like a description of a kidney area rather than of an adrenal zone.)

Aldosterone stimulates sodium reabsorption in the late distal tubules and collecting ducts[1] (the reader is reminded once more that "late distal tubule" refers to the initial collecting tubule and, possibly, to the connecting segment as well). An action on these late portions of the nephron is just what one would expect for a fine-tuning input, since more than 90 percent of the filtered sodium has already been reabsorbed (by the proximal tubule, ascending loop of Henle, and early distal tubule) by the time the late distal tubule is reached. The total quantity of sodium reabsorption dependent upon the influence of aldosterone is approximately 2 percent of the total filtered sodium. Thus, in the complete absence of aldosterone, one would excrete 2 percent of the filtered sodium, whereas in the presence of maximal plasma concentrations of aldosterone, virtually no sodium would be excreted. Two percent of the filtered sodium may, at first thought, seem small, but it is actually very large because of the huge volume of glomerular filtrate:

$$\text{Total filtered NaCl/day} = \text{GFR} \times P_{Na}$$
$$= 180 \text{ L/day} \times 145 \text{ mmol/L}$$
$$= 26,100 \text{ mmol/day}$$

Thus, aldosterone controls the reabsorption of $0.02 \times 26,100$ mmol/day = 522 mmol/day. In terms of sodium chloride, the form in which most

---

[1] As mentioned earlier, the collecting-duct system is not functionally homogenous; aldosterone probably acts only on the cortical collecting tubules, not the medullary ones.

sodium is ingested, this amounts to approximately 30 g NaCl per day, an amount considerably more than the average person eats. Therefore, by reflex variation of plasma concentrations of aldosterone between minimal and maximal, the excretion of sodium can be finely adjusted to the intake so that total body sodium and extracellular volume remain constant.

It is interesting that aldosterone also stimulates sodium transport by other epithelia in the body, namely, by sweat and salivary glands and by the intestine. The net effect is the same as that exerted on the kidney—a reduction in the sodium content of the luminal fluid. Thus, aldosterone is an all-purpose stimulator of sodium retention.

Aldosterone, like other steroids, exerts its effect by entering its target cells, combining with cytosolic receptors, migrating into the nucleus in combination with its receptor, and stimulating synthesis of a particular mRNA. Just which protein this mRNA codes for and how the protein, once formed, enhances sodium transport is far from settled. The most tenable hypothesis at present is that the newly synthesized proteins somehow activate sodium channels in the luminal membrane; this in turn allows greater entry of sodium into the cell, increased cell sodium concentration, and increased "pumping" of sodium by Na-K-dependent ATPase across the basolateral membrane. In this schema, the increased pumping across the basolateral membrane is driven simply by the increased cell sodium concentration. In addition, an increase in the activity of the Na-K-dependent ATPase itself occurs over a longer span of time.

One result of the fact that aldosterone's enhancement of sodium re-absorption requires time (at least 45 min) for protein synthesis is that decreases in sodium excretion that occur within minutes (as, for example, upon standing up) are clearly not due to increased aldosterone.

Control of Aldosterone Secretion   How is aldosterone secretion con-trolled? At least four distinct direct inputs to the adrenal gland are rec-ognized at present (Fig.7-4): (1) plasma sodium concentration, (2) plasma potassium concentration, (3) adrenocorticotropic hormone (ACTH), and (4) angiotensin II.

The first two of these inputs are not mediated by nerves or by hormones. Rather, the adrenal cortex responds to the sodium and potassium concen-trations of the blood perfusing it or to some adrenal intracellular derivative of these concentrations, such as adrenal-cell sodium concentration. This is one of the true "sodium" receptors referred to earlier in this chapter, and the fact that aldosterone secretion is controlled, in part, by plasma sodium concentration makes good sense: Increased plasma sodium → decreased al-dosterone secretion → decreased tubular sodium reabsorption → increased sodium excretion → decreased plasma sodium concentration. However, in humans, this is a very minor control of aldosterone secretion—a fact which

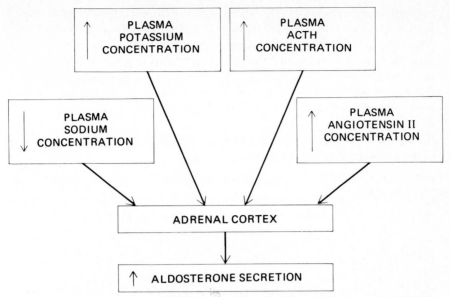

Figure 7-4 Direct controls of aldosterone secretion. A reversal of all arrows in the top boxes would lead to a decrease in aldosterone secretion.

also makes sense teleologically since plasma sodium *concentration* generally changes very little despite marked changes in extracellular *volume*. (Remember that water movements into or out of body cells tend to keep osmolarity and, thereby, plasma sodium concentration, relatively stable.) The influence of plasma potassium concentration on aldosterone secretion is important and will be described in the chapter on renal handling of potassium.

ACTH is the hormone from the anterior pituitary that controls secretion of the other major adrenocortical hormone, cortisol. There is no question that when ACTH is secreted in very large amounts, as during physical trauma, it also stimulates aldosterone secretion. Moreover, even in lower concentrations, ACTH is permissive for other stimulators of aldosterone secretion. Thus, ACTH does play significant roles in the control of aldosterone secretion. However, the secretion of ACTH is not keyed to sodium homeostasis; i.e., it does not usually participate in reflexes specifically "aimed" at maintaining a constant level of body sodium.

We are left with our fourth input, angiotensin II, as the most important known[2] controller of aldosterone secretion in sodium-regulating reflexes. As decribed in Chap. 1, the primary determinant of the plasma concentration of

---

[2] Several groups of investigators have made a strong case for the existence of important but as yet unidentified aldosterone stimulators in addition to the four mentioned here. The pituitary hormones β-endorphin and β-lipotropin, as well as dopamine, are prime candidates.

angiotensin II is the plasma concentration of renin, which is itself determined mainly by the rate of renin secretion. Accordingly, control of aldosterone secretion is, in large part, ultimately determined by those factors which regulate renin secretion (at this point, the reader should review the section on control of renin secretion in Chap. 5). Thus, when plasma volume is reduced by hemorrhage, diarrhea, etc., renin secretion is stimulated, which leads, via angiotensin II, to an increased aldosterone secretion (Fig. 7-5).

Factors Other Than Aldosterone which Influence Tubular Reabsorption of Sodium

Despite its unquestioned primary importance in the regulation of tubular reabsorption of sodium, aldosterone is not the only factor which does so in response to alterations in body sodium balance. Identification of these other factors has been the most investigated subject in renal physiology during the past two decades, but we are still left with great uncertainty concerning the quantitative significance of the many such factors which have been uncovered. Accordingly, one can presently do little more than describe briefly each of the major candidates.

Natriuretic Hormone   The evidence for the existence of a *natriuretic*, or salt-losing, hormone is growing more solid. It suggests that such a hormone is released when extracellular volume is expanded and that it acts upon the tubules to inhibit sodium reabsorption, perhaps by inhibiting Na-K-dependent ATPase. Conversely, one would presume that this hormone's basal secretion would be inhibited when extracellular volume is contracted, with the result that sodium reabsorption by the collecting ducts is enhanced. The site of production of this hypothesized natriuretic hormone is not known, but prime candidates are the cardiac atria (from which can be extracted an *atrial natriuretic factor*) and the brain. The pathways that might control the release of natriuretic hormone are also not known.

Intrarenal Physical Factors: Interstitial Hydraulic Pressure   A factor which can influence net fluid reabsorption is the hydraulic pressure in the renal interstitium. Recall from the previous chapter that although interstitial hydraulic pressure is one of the forces favoring the last step in fluid reabsorption — movement into the peritubular capillaries — it also constitutes an important force simultaneously driving fluid back into the tubular lumen across the tight junctions between cells. This back-leakage, of course, reduces *net* tubular fluid reabsorption, i.e., "short circuits" some of the reabsorption achieved by the forces moving sodium, chloride, and water out of the lumen into the interstitium. The important generalization then is: Whenever interstitial hydraulic pressure is elevated, there is a tendency

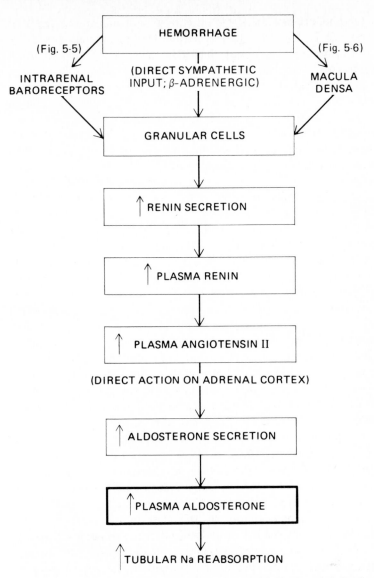

Figure 7-5 Pathway by which aldosterone secretion is increased during hemorrhage.

for overall fluid reabsorption to be decreased (because of increased back-leakage). This is true not only for sodium, chloride, and water but for almost all solutes reabsorbed proximally, the major site of influence by interstitial hydraulic pressure, since the back-leakage involves bulk flow of all interstitial contents. Conversely, a decrease in interstitial hydraulic pressure favors fluid reabsorption (because back-leakage is diminished).

The factors that are most important in setting the steady-state interstitial hydraulic pressure in the kidneys are really the same as in any other location in the body—the capillary hydraulic and oncotic pressures — since these are the dominant forces determining the steady-state volume of fluid in the interstitium. An increased hydraulic pressure inside the capillary tends to raise interstitial hydraulic pressure by causing fluid to accumulate in the interstitium; a decrease in plasma oncotic pressure does precisely the same. Therefore, via its effects on interstitial hydraulic pressure and back-leakage into the tubular lumen, increased hydraulic pressure in the peritubular capillaries reduces tubular fluid reabsorption. Conversely, decreased peritubular-capillary hydraulic pressure facilitates reabsorption. An increased oncotic pressure in peritubular capillaries also facilitates reabsorption, whereas a decreased oncotic pressure reduces reabsorption. Thus, earlier in this chapter we saw that changes in *glomerular-capillary* hydraulic and oncotic pressures were controlled so as to regulate GFR and, thereby, sodium excretion; now we see that analogous changes in the *peritubular-capillary* hydraulic and oncotic pressures help regulate sodium reabsorption and, thereby, sodium excretion.[3]

Teleologically, it makes good sense that such changes in these intra-renal *physical factors* regulate sodium balance and extracellular volume by altering sodium reabsorption. Volume depletion (as in our example of diarrhea) causes decreased peritubular-capillary hydraulic pressure (just as it does decreased glomerular-capillary hydraulic pressure) because of reduced arterial pressure and reflex renal vasoconstriction (Fig.7-6), as well as decreased venous pressure. The effect of the reduced pressure is to enhance sodium reabsorption. The sodium depletion also causes concentration of plasma protein, and this increased oncotic pressure also enhances tubular sodium reabsorption, just as it reduces GFR.

In the last example above, the change in peritubular-capillary oncotic pressure simply reflects a change in systemic-plasma oncotic pressure. Now, we introduce a new but predictable fact: Peritubular-capillary oncotic pressure can be changed independently of any changes in systemic oncotic pressure. The information needed to understand this phenonmenon has already been given: Peritubular-capillary oncotic pressure *always* differs from systemic oncotic pressure, since the plasma proteins are concentrated by loss of protein-free filtrate during passage through the glomerular capillaries. The degree of oncotic-pressure increase depends upon the fraction of the renal plasma flow that is filtered at the glomerulus; this *filtration fraction* is not always the same but varies depending upon the distribution of renal arteriolar constriction. Recall from Chap. 5 that reflex vasoconstriction me-

---

[3] There may also be mechanisms other than back-leakage by which peritubular physical factors influence sodium reabsorption. (See Suggested Readings.)

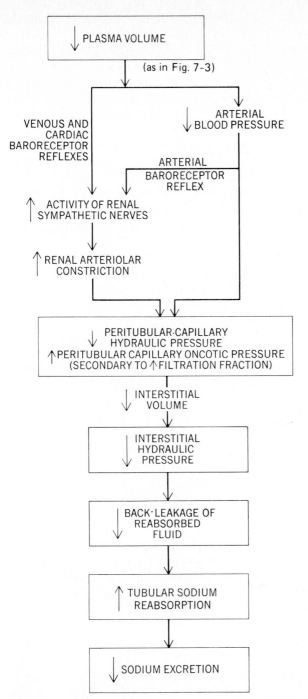

Figure 7-6 Pathway by which changes in intrarenal physical factors are elicited by changes in plasma volume. Compare this to Fig. 7-3, the figure for GFR control; clearly the same inputs that tend to lower GFR also tend to increase sodium reabsorption. As with Fig. 7-3, for simplicity, circulating catecholamines and the renin-angiotensin system have not been included.

diated either by the renal nerves or by circulating agents generally affects not only the afferent arterioles but the efferent ones as well. The net result is that both GFR and RPF decrease but the latter more than the former; therefore, the filtration fraction, GFR/RPF, increases. Accordingly, there occurs a larger-than-normal increase in peritubular-capillary oncotic pressure, and an increased reabsorption of sodium. Conversely, reflexly induced renal vasodilation (as might occur after increased ingestion of salt and water) would be associated with a decreased filtration fraction, a smaller-than-normal rise in peritubular-capillary oncotic pressure, and less sodium reabsorption. Thus, the filtration fraction, by altering peritubular-capillary oncotic pressure, is a determinant of sodium reabsorption.

Just how important are these physical factors in the normal control of sodium and water reabsorption? As might be predicted from information given in Chap. 6, their influence is seen mainly in the proximal tubule, since only this nephron segment has tight junctions leaky enough to permit much back-leakage of fluid. There seems little question that when alterations in fluid balance are very large (as, for example, during severe hemorrhage), proximal reabsorption does change mainly because of the large alterations in the physical factors we have been discussing. Whether significant changes in proximal reabsorption occur in response to more modest alterations in fluid balance (as might result, for example, from eating a diet very low or very high in sodium chloride) is still not known for certain.

Redistribution of Renal Blood Flow   Another potential mechanism for altering sodium excretion is *redistribution of renal blood flow*. It has been hypothesized that certain nephrons may have less capacity to reabsorb sodium than others. Were this true, then at any given total GFR, the relative amounts of fluid filtered by the two different nephron populations would be an important determinant of sodium excretion. Specifically, a redistribution of GFRs to the "high-reabsorption" nephrons, secondary, say, to altered sympathetic input to the two populations, would be associated with decreased sodium excretion because of the greater capacity of these nephrons to reabsorb sodium. Moreover, one can also imagine a redistribution of RPF out of proportion to that of GFR so that filtration fraction and, thereby, fluid reabsorption, could be enhanced in certain nephrons with no change in total renal RPF. Despite the attractiveness of these theories, the evidence in favor of them has not yet been very convincing.

Direct Tubular Effects of Catecholamines   Preceding sections have detailed how the renal sympathetic nerves and circulating epinephrine can influence sodium reabsorption by altering not only renin secretion but also intrarenal physical factors. In this section, we now emphasize that these inputs also stimulate sodium reabsorption by a *direct* action on the tubular cells themselves. (There are numerous neuron terminals adjacent to tubular cells.) The proximal tubule is one site affected by this direct input (which has the same adaptive significance as the indirect renal effects of altered sympathetic activity), but whether other segments are also involved and what type of adrenergic receptor is involved are not yet clear.

Direct Tubular Effects of Angiotensin II   This story reads almost identically to the previous paragraph. Angiotensin II enhances sodium reabsorption indirectly both through its stimulation of aldosterone and its effects on intrarenal physical factors. (Recall that angiotensin II constricts renal arterioles and raises filtration fraction.) In addition, it seems to act directly on the renal cells themselves to stimulate sodium reabsorption.[4] Again, as is the case with the catecholamines, the proximal tubule is involved in this direct response, but other nephron segments may be as well.

We have been chewing at the effects of angiotensin II in small bites throughout this book, and this seems an appropriate place to digest them as well as to gulp down those remaining. The fact is that angiotensin II exerts a bewildering array of effects on many bodily sites, but the common denominator of those with which we are concerned is that they all favor salt retention and elevation of arterial blood pressure. Figure 7-7 summarizes these, adding the facts, not previously mentioned, that angiotensin II stimulates ADH secretion and thirst and facilitates the activity of the sympathetic nervous system. It is crucial to recognize that when renin secretion is elevated in response to physiological stimuli, such as sodium deprivation, all the effects of angiotensin II shown in Fig. 7-7 serve to minimize fluid depletion and to prevent blood pressure from falling below normal. In contrast, when either a *primary* or inappropriate increase in renin secretion occurs due to disease (as in renal artery stenosis, for example), these effects will tend to elevate the blood pressure above normal.

Other Known Humoral Agents   Cortisol, estrogen, growth hormone, and insulin are all known to enhance sodium reabsorption, whereas glucagon, progesterone, and parathyroid hormone all decrease it. It is almost certain that when the level of any of these hormones is elevated (as, for example, estrogen during pregnancy), it will exert a significant influence on sodium reabsorption and, thereby, excretion. However, there is no reason to believe that any of them, unlike the factors described previously, are reflexly controlled specifically so as to homeostatically regulate sodium balance.

---

[4] A source of considerable potential confusion is the fact that angiotensin II, when present in extremely high ("pharmacological") amounts, inhibits sodium reabsorption rather than stimulating it.

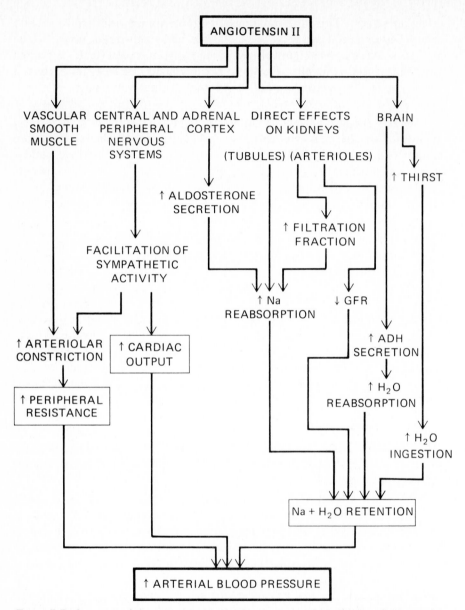

Figure 7-7 Summary of those angiotensin-mediated actions which facilitate fluid retention and elevate the arterial blood pressure. The arrow connecting "Na and H_2O retention" to "arterial blood pressure" is a shortcut for the sake of simplicity—of course, fluid retention influences arterial blood pressure only by altering cardiac output and peripheral resistance. The effects shown in this figure have all been documented for angiotensin II; some may also be exerted by angiotensin III.

Also of great interest is the possible role played by intrarenal humoral systems, particularly the prostaglandins, the kinins, and dopamine. These agents are known to be able to reduce sodium reabsorption by altering intrarenal physical factors (as we have seen, they are potent vasodilators) and/or by direct actions on the tubular cells. Their concentrations are also known to change with alterations of sodium balance, but it is not yet possible to integrate these systems with any assurance into the overall picture of renal sodium regulation.[5]

SUMMARY OF THE CONTROL OF SODIUM EXCRETION

The control of sodium excretion depends mainly upon the control of two variables of renal function, the GFR and the rate of sodium reabsorption (Table 7-2). The latter is controlled most importantly by the renin-angiotensin-aldosterone hormone system, but also by the sympathetic nervous system and several other less well defined factors. The last category probably includes changes in intrarenal hydraulic and oncotic pressures (the so-called physical factors), a natriuretic (or salt-losing) hormone, and, possibly, the distribution of blood flow within the kidney. The renal sympathetic nerves play a prominent role in each of the following: control of aldosterone via renin-angiotensin, determination of intrarenal physical factors, the reabsorptive activity of the tubular cells themselves, and the control of GFR. Yet because of the many other known (and unknown) factors involved, a transplanted and, therefore, denervated kidney maintains sodium homeostasis quite well.

The reflexes that control both GFR and sodium reabsorption are essentially blood-pressure-regulating reflexes, since they are probably most frequently initiated by changes in arterial or venous pressure. This is fitting, since cardiovascular function depends upon an adequate plasma volume, which, as a component of the extracellular-fluid volume, normally reflects the mass of sodium in the body. In normal persons, these regulatory mechanisms are so precise that sodium balance does not vary by more than 2 percent despite marked changes in dietary intake or losses due to sweating, vomiting, diarrhea, hemorrhage, or burns.

---

[5] One suspected role of the prostaglandins in controlling sodium excretion is analogous to their modulating effects on renal hemodynamics (Chap. 5) and water reabsorption (Chap. 6); i.e., they partially offset the effects of substances with opposite actions. During salt depletion, as we have seen, a variety of inputs stimulate sodium reabsorption; simultaneously several of these (sympathetic activity and angiotensin II) induce the release of prostaglandins (Chap. 5). These prostaglandins inhibit sodium reabsorption, thereby causing more sodium to be excreted than would otherwise have been. This helps explain why some persons receiving inhibitors of prostaglandin synthesis manifest inadequate sodium excretion and, hence, sodium retention leading to edema.

Table 7-2   Changes in These Factors Regulate Sodium Excretion in Response to Changes in Extracellular Volume

---

Filtration of sodium
  *GFR
  *Plasma sodium concentration (of minor importance except in severe disorders)

Tubular reabsorption of sodium
  *GFR
  *Aldosterone
  *Intrarenal "physical factors"
  *Renal nerves and circulating epinephrine (direct tubular effects)
  Natriuretic hormone
  *Angiotensin II (direct tubular effects)
  Prostaglandins, kinins, and dopamine
  Distribution of GFRs to different nephrons

---

*Asterisks denote factors for whose participation the evidence is very strong. Roles for the others are likely but have not been conclusively documented. Not listed in the table are hormones that can influence sodium excretion but that are probably not homeostatically controlled primarily for that "purpose."

In several types of disease, however, sodium balance becomes deranged by the failure of the kidneys to excrete sodium normally. Sodium excretion may fall virtually to zero and remain there despite continued sodium ingestion, and the patient retains large quantities of sodium and water within the body, leading to abnormal expansion of extracellular fluid and formation of edema. An important example of this phenomenon is congestive heart failure. A patient with a failing heart (i.e., a heart whose contractility is too low to maintain the cardiac output required for the body's metabolic requirements) usually manifests decreased GFR and increased activity of the renin-angiotensin-aldosterone system. In addition, renal filtration fraction is almost always increased—a situation that causes increased oncotic pressure in the peritubular capillaries. All these, and perhaps other sodium-retaining factors, contribute to the almost complete reabsorption of sodium. The net result is expansion of plasma volume, increased capillary pressure, and filtration of fluid into the interstitial space (edema).

Why do these sodium-retaining reflexes continue to be elicited despite the fact that the person is in markedly positive and progressively increasing sodium balance? The answer stems from the fact, described earlier, that total extracellular volume itself is not directly monitored. In the normal person there is no discrepancy between changes in total extracellular volume and total body sodium, on the one hand, and plasma volume, cardiovascular pressures, and cardiac output, on the other. Thus, a reflex triggered by a change in these latter derivative functions will end up homeostatically regulating body sodium and extracellular volume. In contrast, because of a failing heart, there is a discontinuity between these two groups of variables; i.e., the patient has an inadequate cardiac output despite an increased extracellular volume. This reduced cardiac output initiates, most likely via arterial baroreceptors (which reduce their firing rates because of the decrease in mean and pulsatile arterial pressure),[6] sodium-retaining reflexes just as would occur in a normal person whose cardiac output had been reduced due to hemorrhage or severe diarrhea.

There are several other conditions, specifically the liver disease cirrhosis and the kidney syndrome nephrosis, that tend to produce sodium retention of this kind. They, too, are characterized by persistent sodium-retaining reflexes (decreased GFR, increased aldosterone, etc.) despite progressive overexpansion of extracellular fluid and formation of edema, as in congestive heart failure. All these edematous conditions, including congestive heart failure, are sometimes called diseases of *secondary hyperaldosteronism* because they are usually associated with increased secretion of aldosterone *secondary* to increased renin, which in turn is due to the inappropriate reflexes just described.

At one time it was thought that the elevated aldosterone was sufficient in itself to cause progressive accumulation of sodium. It is now recognized that such is not the case and that one or more of the other factors that influence sodium excretion must also be operating to maintain the retention. This is nicely illustrated by the difference in sodium handling between *primary hyperaldosteronism* and the diseases of secondary hyperaldosteronism. Primary hyperaldosteronism is characterized by persistent oversecretion of aldosterone due to a primary adrenal defect, usually an aldosterone-producing tumor. Because of the increased aldosterone, sodium retention does occur *initially*, but after a few days, there occurs an *escape* from the effects of aldosterone, i.e., a return to normal sodium excretion despite the continued presence of increased aldosterone. (After balance is reestablished, a persistent, small, positive sodium balance does remain.) What has happened is that the initial sodium retention causes expansion of extracellular volume and total body sodium, which then initiates sodium-losing responses: (1) GFR often rises; and (2) the factors (e.g., natriuretic hormone and renal physical factors) other than aldosterone that act on the tubule change so as to reduce sodium reabsorption (mainly upstream from the collecting ducts). The net effect of these responses is to supply so much sodium to the collecting ducts that, despite hyperreabsorption in this segment (under the influence of the excess aldosterone) sodium excretion is restored to normal.

---

[6] In addition, baroreceptors in the great veins and cardiac chambers appear to be damaged by (or adapted to) the engorgement occurring in these locations and manifest decreased rates of firing despite the marked degree of distention.

In other words, persistent, progressive sodium retention cannot be induced by an abnormality in only one of the factors controlling sodium excretion, since reflexes will rapidly be induced whereby opposing changes in the other factors will restore normal sodium excretion. Only when essentially all inputs are altering sodium excretion, either appropriately, as in sodium depletion, or inappropriately, as in the diseases of secondary hyperaldosteronism with edema, will sodium excretion remain continuously near zero; in these latter diseases, "escape" does not occur from the effects of persistently elevated aldosterone.

ADH SECRETION AND EXTRACELLULAR VOLUME

Although we have spoken of extracellular-volume regulation only in terms of the control of sodium excretion, it is clear that, to be most effective in altering extracellular volume, the changes in sodium excretion must be accompanied by equivalent changes in water excretion. We have already pointed out that the ability of water to follow when sodium is reabsorbed depends upon ADH. Accordingly, it is critical that a decreased extracellular volume reflexly call forth increased ADH production as well as increased aldosterone secretion. What is the nature of this reflex? ADH is an octapeptide produced by a discrete group of hypothalamic neurons whose cell bodies are located in the supraoptic and paraventricular nuclei and whose axons terminate in the posterior pituitary, from which ADH is released into the blood. These hypothalamic cells receive input from venous, cardiac and arterial baroreceptors, particularly those located in the left atrium (Fig. 7-8). The baroreceptors are stimulated by increased atrial blood pressure, and the impulses resulting from this stimulation are transmitted via afferent nerves and ascending pathways to the hypothalamus, where they inhibit the ADH-producing cells. Conversely, decreased atrial pressure causes less firing by the baroreceptors and a resulting stimulation of ADH synthesis and release (Fig. 7-9). The adaptive value of this baroreceptor reflex is to help restore extracellular volume and, hence, blood pressure.

There is a second adaptive value to this reflex: Large decreases in extracellular volume elicit, by way of the cardiovascular baroreceptors, such high concentrations of ADH that the hormone is able to exert direct vasoconstrictor effects on arteriolar smooth muscle; the result is an increased total peripheral resistance, which helps raise arterial blood pressure independently of the more slowly occurring restoration of body-fluid volumes. Renal arterioles (and mesangial cells) participate in this constrictor response, and so a high plasma concentration of ADH, quite apart from

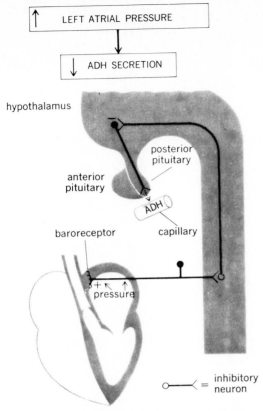

Figure 7-8 Major pathway by which ADH secretion is decreased when plasma volume is increased. The greater plasma volume raises left atrial pressure, which stimulates the atrial baroreceptors and inhibits ADH secretion. Other baroreceptors also participate in this reflex. (*From A. J. Vander et al., Human Physiology,* © *1970 by McGraw-Hill, Inc. Used with permission of McGraw-Hill Book Company.*)

its effect on tubular water permeability, may promote retention of both sodium and water by lowering GFR.

As shown in Fig. 7-7, angiotensin II also stimulates ADH release, just as it does aldosterone secretion. Thus, the renin-angiotensin system may play a role in enhancing water reabsorption (via ADH) as it does sodium (via aldosterone), but the quantitative importance of this pathway is much less than that of the atrial baroreceptor reflex for ADH just described.

ADH AND THE RENAL REGULATION OF EXTRACELLULAR OSMOLARITY

We turn now to the renal compensation for pure-water losses or gains, e.g., the situation in which a person drinks 2 L of water, but no change in the

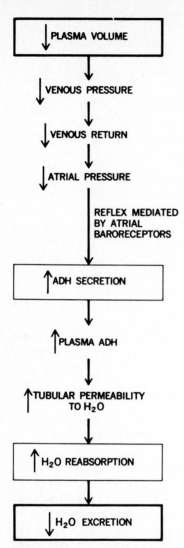

Figure 7-9 Major pathway by which ADH secretion is increased when plasma volume decreases. This figure is merely the converse of Fig. 7-8. (*From A. J. Vander et al., Human Physiology, © 1970 by McGraw-Hill, Inc. Used with permission of McGraw-Hill Book Company.*)

total bodily salt content occurs. Only the total water changes. The most efficient compensatory mechanism is for the kidneys to excrete the excess water without altering its usual excretion of salt, and this is precisely what they do. ADH secretion is reflexly inhibited, as will be described below; water permeability of the more distal segments of the nephron becomes very low; sodium reabsorption proceeds normally but water is unable to follow; and a large volume of extremely dilute urine is excreted. In this manner, the excess pure water is eliminated. Conversely, when a pure-water deficit occurs, ADH secretion is reflexly stimulated, water permeability of these segments is increased, water reabsorption occurs at a maximal rate, the final urine volume becomes extremely small, and its osmolarity is considerably greater than that of the plasma. By this means, relatively less of the filtered water than solute is excreted—which is equivalent to adding pure water to the body—and the pure-water deficit is compensated.

The renal contribution to alterations in body-fluid osmolarity is quantifiable through use of a term known as the *clearance of solute-free water*, abbreviated C_{H_2O}. Note immediately that the term is not *water* clearance, which would denote, by conventional clearance terminology, the volume of water removed from the plasma per unit time. Instead, free-water clearance is not really a true clearance at all but denotes the volume of *pure water* which would have to be either removed from or added to the urine to make it isoosmotic to plasma. Let us take as an example the excretion of 1 L of urine per day, having an osmolarity of 150 mosmol/L. Now, imagine that this liter of urine really consists of 500 mL of isoosmotic fluid (300 mosmol/L) and 500 mL of pure water; accordingly, the free-water clearance in this case is 500 mL, and this is the volume of pure water eliminated from the body. Another example—1 L of urine having an osmolarity of 1200 mosmol/L. Three liters of pure water would have to be *added* to this liter to make it isoosmotic; in terms of the body-fluid osmolarity, excretion of this liter of urine, therefore, has essentially the same effect as if 3 L of pure water had been added to the body. In essence, this is just what the collecting ducts did by reabsorbing 3 L of water without accompanying solute. Whenever the urine is hypoosmotic, free-water clearance is said to be "positive"; when it is hyperosmotic, free-water clearance is said to be "negative." A positive free-water clearance denotes the excretion of free water, whereas a negative free-water clearance denotes the reabsorption of free water. Therefore, an appropriate synonym for negative free-water clearance is the symbol $T^C_{H_2O}$, which stands for "the volume of free water reabsorbed (transported, T) by the collecting ducts (superscript C)."

The formula for calculating free-water clearance is as follows:

$$C_{H_2O} = V - \frac{U_{osmol}V}{P_{osmol}}$$

where V is the urine volume per unit time, U_{osmol} is the urine osmolarity, and P_{osmol} is the plasma osmolarity (the formula was not given initially so that the reader would be forced to deal with the concepts underlying the equation). Thus, in our examples above:

$$C_{H_2O} = 1 \text{ L/day} - \frac{150 \text{ mOsm/L} \cdot 1 \text{ L/day}}{300 \text{ mOsm/L}} = 0.5 \text{ L/day}$$

$$C_{H_2O} = 1 \text{ L/day} - \frac{1200 \text{ mOsm/L} \cdot 1 \text{ L/day}}{300 \text{ mOsm/L}} = -3.0 \text{ L/day}$$

To reiterate, pure-water deficits or gains are compensated by partially dissociating water excretion from that of salt through changes in ADH secretion. What receptor input controls ADH under such conditions? The answer is: changes in body-fluid osmolarity. The adaptive rationale should be obvious, since osmolarity is the variable most affected by pure-water gains or deficits. The osmoreceptors involved are located in the hypothalamus, the liver, and probably other sites as well; the mechanism by which they detect changes in osmolarity is unknown.[7] The hypothalamic cells which secrete ADH receive neural input from these osmoreceptors. Via these connections, an increase in osmolarity stimulates them and increases their rate of ADH secretion; conversely, decreased osmolarity inhibits ADH secretion (Fig. 7-10). The osmoreceptors are extraordinarily sensitive: for example, a 1% decrease in osmolarity (producible by drinking less than 500 ml of water) suffices to trigger, via the osmoreceptors, a reduction in ADH secretion adequate to increase water excretion.

We have now described two different major afferent pathways controlling the ADH-secreting hypothalamic cells, one from baroreceptors and one from osmoreceptors. These hypothalamic cells are, therefore, true integrating centers whose rate of activity is determined by the total synaptic input. Thus, a simultaneous increase in extracellular volume and decrease in extracellular osmolarity causes strong inhibition of ADH secretion; conversely, the opposite changes produce marked stimulation (there seems to be a synergism between these two inputs). But what happens when baroreceptor and osmoreceptor inputs oppose each other, as for example if extracellular volume and osmolarity are both decreased? In general, the osmoreceptor influence predominates over that of the baroreceptor when changes in osmolarity and extracellular volume are small to moderate, because of the greater sensitivity of the osmoreceptors. However, a very large change in

---

[7] Some evidence suggests that these receptors may actually be sensitive to sodium rather than to osmolarity. The end result is the same, since sodium is normally the major determinant of osmolarity. Of clinical interest is the fact that the receptors are not affected by changes in plasma urea or glucose; accordingly, the increases in these substances in uremia and diabetes mellitus, respectively, will not increase ADH secretion.

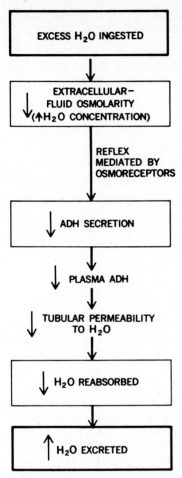

Figure 7-10 Pathway by which ADH secretion is lowered and water excretion raised when excess water is ingested. *(From A. J. Vander et al., Human Physiology, © 1970 by McGraw-Hill, Inc. Used with permission of McGraw-Hill Book Company.)*

extracellular volume will take precedence over osmolarity in influencing ADH secretion.

To add to the complexity, the ADH-secreting cells respond, as we have seen, to angiotensin II, and they also receive synaptic input from many other brain areas; thus, ADH secretion and, therfore, urine flow can be altered by pain, fear, and a variety of other factors. However, these effects are usually short-lived and should not obscure the generalization that ADH secretion is determined primarily by the states of extracellular volume and osmolarity. Alcohol is a powerful inhibitor of ADH release—a fact that probably accounts for much of the large urine flow accompanying the ingestion of alcohol.

The disease diabetes insipidus, which is different from diabetes mellitus, or sugar diabetes, illustrates what happens when the ADH system is disrupted. Diabetes insipidus is characterized by the constant excretion of a large volume of highly dilute urine (as much as 25 L/day). In most cases, the flow can be restored to normal by the administration of ADH. These patients apparently have lost the ability to produce ADH, usually as a result of damage to the hypothalamus. Thus, late distal-tubule and collecting-duct permeability to water is low and unchanging regardless of extracellular osmolarity or volume. The very thought of having to urinate (and therefore to drink) 25 L of water per day underscores the importance of ADH in the control of renal function and body-water balance. In contrast, other diseases are associated with inappropriately large secretion of ADH. As is predictable, patients with these diseases manifest a decreased plasma osmolarity because of the excessive reabsorption of pure water.

Figure 7-11 summarizes many of the factors known to control renal sodium and water reabsorption in response to severe sweating, as in exercise.

THIRST AND SALT APPETITE

Now we must turn to the other component of the balance — control of intake. It should be evident that large deficits of salt and water can be only partly compensated by renal conservation and that ingestion is the ultimate compensatory mechanism. The subjective feeling of thirst, which drives one to obtain and ingest water, is stimulated both by a reduced extracellular volume and by an increased plasma osmolarity. The adaptive significance of both are self-evident. Note that these are precisely the same changes that stimulate ADH production. The centers that mediate thirst are located in the hypothalamus and are very close to those areas that produce ADH. They are also very close to, but distinct from, food-intake centers. Damage to the thirst centers completely abolishes the drive for water intake. Conversely, electric stimulation of them may induce profound and prolonged drinking.

Because of the similarities between the stimuli for ADH secretion and for thirst, it is tempting to speculate that the receptors (osmoreceptors and atrial baroreceptors) that initiate the ADH-controlling reflexes are identical to those for thirst. This may, indeed, be the case, but there are also other pathways controlling thirst. For example, dryness of the mouth and throat causes profound thirst, which is relieved by merely moistening them. It is fascinating that when animals such as the camel (and humans, to a lesser extent) become markedly dehydrated, they will rapidly drink just enough

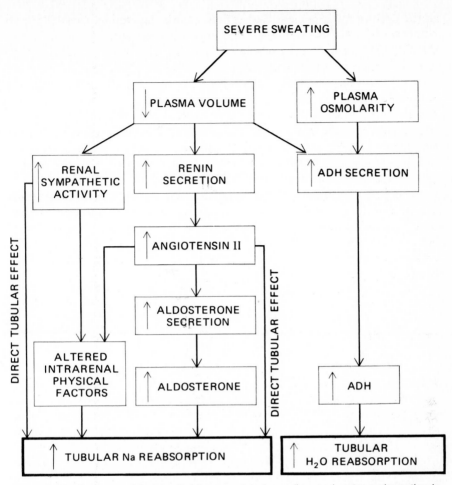

Figure 7-11 Summary of factors that increase tubular sodium and water reabsorption in severe sweating. These changes, coupled with the decrease in GFR which also occurs, homeostatically reduce urinary sodium and water loss.

water to replace their previous losses and then stop. What is amazing is that when they stop, the water has not yet had time to be absorbed from the gastrointestinal tract into the blood. Some kind of metering of the water intake by the gastrointestinal tract has occurred, but its nature remains a mystery.

As shown in Fig. 7-7, angiotensin II stimulates thirst by a direct effect on the brain and constitutes one of the pathways by which thirst is stimulated when extracellular volume is decreased.

Salt appetite, which is the analogue of thirst, is also an extremely important component of sodium homeostasis in most mammals, particularly in the herbivores. It is clear that salt appetite is innate and consists of two components: hedonistic appetite and regulatory appetite. In other words, animals like salt and eat it whenever they can, regardless of whether they are salt-deficient, and, in addition, their drive to obtain salt is markedly increased in the presence of deficiency. The significance of these animal studies for humans is unclear. Salt craving does seem to occur in humans who are severely salt-depleted, but the contribution of regulatory salt appetite to everyday sodium homeostasis in normal persons is probably slight. On the other hand, humans do seem to have a strong hedonistic appetite for salt, as manifested by almost universally large intakes of sodium whenever it is cheap and readily available. Thus, the average American intake of salt is 10 to 15 g/day despite the fact that humans can survive quite normally on less than 0.5 g/day. Present evidence suggests that a large salt intake may be a contributor to the pathogenesis of hypertension.

Study questions: 44 to 59

CHAPTER 8

RENAL REGULATION OF POTASSIUM BALANCE

OBJECTIVES

The student understands the internal exchanges of potassium.

1 States the normal distribution of body potassium
2 States the effects of epinephrine, insulin, aldosterone, acidosis, and alkalosis on potassium movement into cells

The student understands the renal regulation of potassium.

1 Describes the basic renal processes for handling potassium in each nephron segment, including medullary cycling
2 Contrasts the contribution of each nephron site to potassium handling during a high- and low-potassium diet
3 Describes the mechanism by which potassium secretion is accomplished by the distal nephron
4 Lists the inputs that control the rate of potassium secretion by the distal nephron so as to regulate potassium balance homeostatically; defines potassium adaptation
5 Describes the pathway by which changes in potassium balance influence aldosterone secretion
6 Describes the effects of alkalosis on potassium secretion and balance
7 Describes the relationship between renal sodium handling, diuretics, and potassium secretion; contrasts distal-tubular secretion of potassium in persons with primary versus secondary hyperaldosteronism
8 Predicts the changes in potassium excretion and balance occurring in representative abnormal situations: respiratory or metabolic alkalosis, primary aldosteronism, diarrhea, diabetes mellitus

The potassium concentration of the extracellular fluid is a closely regulated quantity. The importance of maintaining this concentration in the internal environment stems primarily from the role of potassium in the excitability of nerve and muscle. The resting membrane potentials of these tissues are directly related to the ratio of intracellular to extracellular potassium concentration. Raising the external potassium concentration lowers the resting membrane potential, thus increasing cell excitability. Conversely, lowering the external potassium hyperpolarizes cell membranes and reduces their excitability.

Extracellular potassium concentration is a function of two variables: (1) the total amount of potassium in the body; (2) the distribution of this potassium between the extracellular and intracellular fluid compartments. The first variable, total body potassium, is determined by the relative rates of potassium intake and excretion. Normal individuals remain in potassium balance (as they do in sodium balance) by excreting daily an amount of potassium equal to the amount of potassium ingested minus the small amounts eliminated in the feces and sweat. Normally, potassium losses via sweat and the gastrointestinal tract are small, although large quantities can be lost by the latter during vomiting or diarrhea. Again, the control of renal function is the major mechanism by which total body potassium is regulated.

However, before describing the renal handling of potassium, we must briefly summarize the less well understood but very important second variable noted above — the distribution of total body potassium between the extracellular and intracellular fluid compartments and the homeostatic regulation of this distribution.

REGULATION OF INTERNAL POTASSIUM DISTRIBUTION

Approximately 98 percent of total body potassium is located within cells because of the Na-K-dependent ATPase plasma-membrane pumps, which actively transport potassium into most cells. Since the amount of potassium in the extracellular compartment is so small, compared to that inside cells, even very small shifts of potassium into or out of cells can produce large changes in extracellular potassium concentration. Such shifts (particularly in muscle and liver) are, to some extent, under physiological control, so that when extracellular potassium concentration changes because of changes either in total body potassium (i.e., imbalances between intake and excretion), or internal shifts secondary to other events (cell damage, for example), potassium moves into or out of cells, thereby minimizing the changes in extracellular concentration. The major factors involved in these homeostatic processes are epinephrine, insulin, and aldosterone.

Epinephrine causes increased net movement of potassium into cells (particularly muscle and liver). This effect is mediated by beta-adrenergic receptors, but the mechanism underlying the net movement is not known. This effect is probably of greatest importance during exercise and trauma. Both these situations are associated with movement of potassium out of certain cells (the exercising muscle cells or the damaged cells); however, they are also associated with increased adrenomedullary secretion of epinephrine, and this hormone's stimulation of potassium uptake partially offsets the outflow occurring from the exercising or damaged cells.

Insulin, at physiological concentrations, exerts a tonic permissive effect promoting net movement of potassium into muscle, liver, and other tissues. Moreover, a very large increase in plasma potassium concentration stimulates insulin secretion, and the additional insulin induces greater potassium uptake by cells.

Aldosterone is also involved in internal potassium exchanges, but its precise contribution is not clear. In general, it seems to facilitate net potassium movement into cells when plasma potassium is chronically elevated because of increased total body potassium content. This action of aldosterone is quite independent of this hormone's effect on renal potassium handling.

Thus far, the discussion has dealt with factors that homeostatically regulate internal potassium movements so as to minimize changes in extracellular potassium concentration. However, there are other factors that can influence potassium movements into or out of cells, but are not homeostatic mechanisms for regulating extracellular potassium; instead they may markedly displace extracellular potassium concentration away from normal. The most important of these is the hydrogen-ion concentration of the body fluids: an increase in hydrogen-ion concentration (acidosis) is often associated with net potassium movement out of cells, and alkalosis with net potassium movement into them.[1] It is as though potassium and hydrogen ions were "exchanging" across the cell membrane (i.e., hydrogen ions moving into the cell during acidosis and out during alkalosis, with potassium doing just the opposite), but the precise mechanism underlying these "exchanges" has not yet been clarified.

BASIC RENAL MECHANISMS

Potassium is completely filterable at the glomerulus.[2] The amounts of

---

[1] There are many exceptions to these generalizations. (See the article by Adrogue and Madias in Suggested Readings.)

[2] Recent evidence suggests that, at least in some species, approximately 10 percent of plasma potassium may actually be protein-bound, but this is not yet generally accepted for human beings.

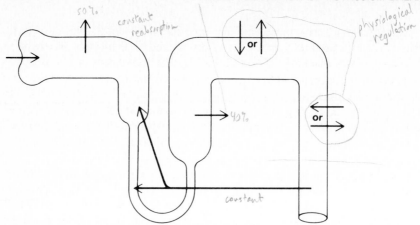

Figure 8-1 Handling of potassium by different nephron segments. Filtration occurs at the glomeruli, and all subsequent arrows denote net tubular reabsorption or secretion. See text for discussion of each segment.

potassium excreted in the urine are generally a small fraction (10 to 15 percent) of the filtered quantity. These facts establish the existence of tubular potassium reabsorption. However, it has also been demonstrated that under certain conditions the excreted quantity may actually exceed the filtered quantity. We therefore conclude that tubular potassium secretion also exists. Thus, the subject is complicated by the fact that potassium can be both reabsorbed and secreted by the tubule. The complexity is further increased because of heterogeneity between short-looped and long-looped nephrons. Let us first follow potassium along the length of a nephron (Fig. 8-1) and then provide several useful simplifying generalizations.

Potassium reabsorption occurs in the proximal convoluted tubule. It is primarily a passive process driven mainly by diffusion,[3] the concentration gradient for which is created (as for urea) by water reabsorption. By the end of the proximal convoluted tubule, approximately 50 percent of the filtered potassium has been reabsorbed.

Then in the straight portion (pars recta) of the proximal tubule and in the descending limb of the loop of Henle, potassium secretion occurs, mainly by passive diffusion down a potassium concentration gradient from interstitium to lumen. (The source of this interstitial potassium will be described in a moment.)

In the ascending limb of Henle's loop, the dominant process for potassium movement is once again passive reabsorption. This is so effective that for short-looped nephrons, the amount of potassium entering the dis-

[3] Some reabsorption is also caused by solvent drag; i.e., the potassium is "dragged" along with the reabsorbed water.

tal convoluted tubule is approximately 10 percent of the mass originally filtered at the glomerulus. In other words, in these nephrons, the proximal convoluted tubule reabsorbs 50 percent of the filtered potassium, and the ascending limb reabsorbs another 40 percent *plus* whatever potassium had been secreted into the pars recta and descending limb. What about the long-looped nephrons? It is likely that here, too, reabsorption along the ascending limb removes from the lumen a large fraction of the potassium that had been present at the bend of the loop, but precisely how much is not known.

To summarize events occurring prior to the distal tubule: Potassium is reabsorbed from both the proximal convoluted tubule and ascending limb, but secreted into the pars recta and descending limb. The reabsorptive processes are greater, so that the amount of potassium entering the distal convoluted tubule is only a fraction of that which was filtered.

Now for the distal tubules and cortical collecting tubules. (The portion of distal tubule involved in potassium transport is the "late" portion — the connecting tubule and initial collecting tubule. The "early" portion — the distal convoluted tubule — plays little, if any role in potassium transport.) The distal tubules and cortical collecting tubules are able both to secrete and to reabsorb potassium, both processes being active (the mechanisms will be described below). The rates at which these opposing processes occur, particularly that of secretion, are variable, depending upon physiological circumstances; accordingly, the *net* contribution of these nephron segments may be either reabsorption or secretion.

Finally, the medullary collecting tubules (and papillary ducts). This segment usually manifests tubular reabsorption[4]; the potassium reabsorbed from this segment is probably the major source of the potassium that is secreted into the pars recta and the descending limb of Henle. Thus, there is a recycling of potassium from the medullary collecting ducts to the straight proximal tubules and descending limbs analagous to that described for urea in Chap. 4.

One might predict that, given the heterogeneity of potassium transport not only between segments of a single nephron but between the several nephron types as well, the control of potassium excretion might be quite complex. However, there are several simplifying generalizations that help a good deal. First, the transport processes in the proximal tubule and loop of Henle are relatively unchanging in the face of increases or decreases in total body potassium; in other words, transport in these nephron segments does not seem to be controlled so as to achieve potassium homeostasis. Accordingly, the amount of potassium reaching the distal tubule is always much less than that which was filtered (despite potassium secretion into the pars recta and

[4] However, under certain circumstances it, too, may be capable of net secretion.

descending limb) and is not physiologically regulated to any great extent. Second (and really a corollary of the first generalization), physiological regulation of potassium excretion is achieved mainly by altering potassium transport in the distal tubule and cortical collecting tubules. The major process regulated in these nephron sites is the rate of potassium secretion.

Let us take a few examples using superficial (short-looped) nephrons, for which micropuncture data are most available; the events for long-looped nephrons would be qualitatively similar. During potassium deprivation (caused, for example, by a low-potassium diet), the homeostatic response is to reduce potassium excretion to a minimal level. Using micropuncture to evaluate potassium handling by each nephron segment, we would find that the proximal tubule and loop were reabsorbing about 90 percent of the filtered potassium and that the distal tubule and collecting duct together were reabsorbing most of the remaining 10 percent so that very little potassium was excreted. Now we shift to the opposite end of the spectrum and look at the kidneys during a very high potassium diet. In this case the homeostatic response is to excrete large quantities of potassium so as to balance output with intake. Micropuncture reveals that the proximal tubule and the loop are still reabsorbing the same fraction (90 percent) of filtered potassium so that the amount of potassium entering the distal tubule from the loop is not much different from the amount entering it when the individual was on the low-potassium diet. Now, the radical difference appears: The distal tubule manifests net secretion of potassium rather than the net reabsorption seen on the low-potassium diet. Indeed, the quantity of potassium added to the distal lumen by secretion may be greater than the quantity of potassium reabsorbed upstream by the proximal tubule and loop. The fluid then leaves the distal tubule and flows through the cortical collecting tubules, where more potassium is added by secretion. Finally, during flow through the medullary portions of the collecting ducts, some potassium is reabsorbed, so that the mass of potassium excreted is less than that leaving the cortical collecting tubules; i.e., reabsorption of potassium by the medullary collecting duct offsets some of the secretion by the distal tubules and cortical collecting tubules. Despite this, the final result is excretion of more potassium than was filtered, i.e., *net secretion* by the *overall nephron*.

These examples should reinforce the generalization that, normally, the major sites for homeostatic control of renal potassium excretion are the distal portions of the nephron, particularly the distal tubule and cortical collecting tubules, whose contribution can be either net reabsorption or net secretion. As we shall see below, the major controlled variables in these segments are those membrane transport processes that lead to secretion. So dominant are these processes that in describing the control of potassium excretion, we will tend to ignore any contribution of changes in either filtered potassium (GFR $\times$ P_K) or tubular transport proximal to the distal tubule. It must be pointed out, however, that under certain abnormal conditions, potassium reabsorption in the proximal tubule or loop may be decreased and that a large quantity of the potassium excreted may represent filtered potassium which is not reabsorbed. For example, drugs that inhibit sodium reabsorption by the proximal tubule or loop also usually inhibit potassium reabsorption at these sites. Another situation characterized by inhibition of proximal and loop potassium reabsorption is osmotic diuresis. Just as was true for sodium, the presence of an osmotic diuretic interferes with potassium reabsorption; this is one reason for the marked urinary loss of potassium suffered by patients with uncontrolled diabetes mellitus.

MECHANISM OF DISTAL POTASSIUM SECRETION

The presently accepted model for potassium secretion by the distal tubule and cortical collecting tubule (for convenience we will refer to these segments simply as "distal") is illustrated in Fig. 8-2. The critical event (step 1) is the active transport of potassium from interstitial fluid across the basolateral membrane into the cell. This active transport step, which is mediated via the Na-K-ATPase system, creates a very high intracellular potassium concentration so that a concentration gradient exists favoring net potassium diffusion from cell into lumen (2) (and, of course, from cell back into interstitial fluid—[a]; however, movement in this "backward" direction is small because the basolateral membrane is much less permeable to potassium than is the luminal membrane). Note that the concentration gradient across the luminal membrane is opposed by an electrical force (30 mV, cell-negative) which favors net diffusion from lumen to cell. However this opposing electrical force is not as large as the chemical force (the concentration gradient), and the result is net diffusion of potassium into the lumen. The luminal membrane is highly permeable to potassium because it contains a large number of potassium-specific channels.[5] Thus, this model for secretion postulates active transport into the cell at the basolateral membrane and passive exit at the luminal membrane.[6] Clearly, in such a model, activity of the basolateral pump emerges as the dominant force driving overall secretion.

But recall that, in the presence of potassium deficit, these nephron segments can manifest net active tubular reabsorption rather than net tubular

[5] This high luminal permeability is one reason that these distal nephron segments can secrete potassium whereas the proximal tubule and ascending thick limb of Henle, which also contain a basolateral Na-K-dependent ATPase but have a much lower luminal permeability to potassium, cannot.

[6] There may also be some component of active potassium transport from cell into lumen, at least in the cortical collecting tubule.

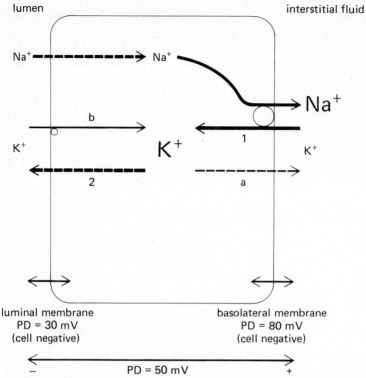

Figure 8-2 Diagrammatic representation of model proposed for distal tubular handling of potassium. As shown here, this cell would be secreting potassium. The dashed lines denote *net* diffusional fluxes across the individual membranes. The numbers and letters serve as guides for the text. The thicknesses of the lines are not drawn to scale; i.e., they serve only to emphasize which flux is greatest at each membrane, not how much greater. Note that the model is based completely on movement of potassium *through cells*, not *between* them; the tight junctions between distal-tubular cells are certainly not completely impermeable to potassium so that some small fraction of potassium secretion probably does occur across them, driven by the favorable potential difference from interstitial fluid to lumen. (This "transtubular" potential difference of 50 mV is, of course, merely the algebraic sum of the luminal and basolateral membrane potentials.) Also not shown in the figure is the likelihood that the reabsorption of potassium (b) requires co-transport with chloride.

secretion. To account for this, the model proposes an active potassium reabsorptive pump[7] in the luminal membrane (b). This pump probably is always operating, albeit at a relatively slow rate, and therefore opposes movement of potassium in the secretory direction; moreover, it will produce net reabsorption whenever the basolateral pump activity is eliminated or greatly reduced. A logical question is whether this luminal reabsorptive pump is itself physiologically regulated—speeded up during potassium deprivation

[7] It is likely that this distal reabsorptive pump somehow requires that chloride be co-transported with the potassium.

and slowed down during potassium excess. The answer to this question is probably yes, but the range of change seems to be small compared to the changes exhibited by the secretory (basolateral) pump, and will be ignored.

To reiterate, potassium secretion requires a cellular accumulation step at the basolateral membrane. This step is best explained by the presence of an active potassium pump (Na-K-ATPase). The elevated intracellular potassium concentration achieved by the basolateral pump is responsible for net diffusion of potassium out of the cell into the lumen. This passive luminal step depends not only on the intracellular potassium concentration achieved by the basolateral pump but on the luminal concentration (the other end of the concentration gradient), the magnitude of the luminal potential difference opposing diffusion into the lumen, and the permeability of the luminal membrane to potassium. How these factors are altered will be described below.

HOMEOSTATIC CONTROL OF DISTAL SECRETION

What are the factors that influence distal potassium secretion so as to achieve homeostasis of body potassium? In other words, how do changes in body potassium induce the kidney to secrete more or less potassium? When a high-potassium diet is ingested (Fig. 8-3), plasma potassium concentration increases, even though very slightly, and this drives enhanced basolateral uptake via the basolateral pump. The resulting increase in intracellular potassium concentration enhances the gradient for potassium movement into the lumen and raises potassium secretion. Conversely, a low-potassium diet or a negative-potassium balance, e.g., from diarrhea, lowers renal-tubular-cell potassium concentration; this reduces potassium secretion and excretion, thereby helping to reestablish potassium balance.

A second important factor linking potassium secretion to potassium balance is the hormone aldosterone, which, besides stimulating tubular sodium reabsorption, simultaneously enhances tubular potassium secretion (Fig. 8-3), in the same nephron segments—late distal tubule and cortical collecting tubule. The reflex by which changes in extracellular volume control aldosterone production is completely different from the reflex initiated by an excess or deficit of potassium. The former constitutes a complex pathway, involving renin and angiotensin II. The latter, however, seems to be much simpler and works in the following way (Fig. 8-3): The aldosterone-secreting cells of the adrenal cortex are apparently sensitive to the potassium concentration of the extracellular fluid bathing them (or, more likely, they are sensitive to their own intracellular potassium concentration). Thus, an increased intake of potassium leads to an increased extracellular potassium concentration, which, in turn, directly stimulates aldosterone production by

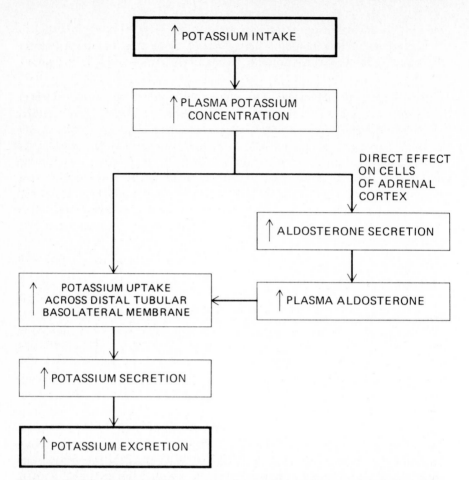

Figure 8-3 Pathways by which an increased potassium intake induces increased potassium excretion. Aldosterone also increases the luminal permeability to potassium. The responsiveness of the renal tubules (i.e., their uptake and secretion of potassium) to increases in plasma potassium and aldosterone is significantly enhanced when the high potassium intake is chronic, an adaptation which reflects an increase in the number of basolateral Na-K-dependent ATPase sites. "Distal" refers to both the distal tubule and cortical collecting tubule.

the adrenal cortex. The resulting increase in plasma aldosterone concentration stimulates potassium secretion by the distal portions of the nephron and, thereby, eliminates the excess potassium from the body.

Aldosterone influences potassium secretion in several ways, but its dominant action is stimulation of the distal basolateral-membrane Na-K-ATPase pumps (Fig. 8-3). (This is consistent with aldosterone's ability to stimulate sodium reabsorption in these same nephron segments.) This increases intracellular potassium concentration and the gradient for movement into the lumen. Aldosterone also increases luminal-membrane permeability to potassium so that the enhanced gradient for diffusion is even more effective in driving luminal entry. Conversely, a lowered extracellular-potassium concentration decreases aldosterone production and, thereby, reduces tubular potassium secretion; less potassium than usual is excreted in the urine, thus helping to restore the normal extracellular potassium concentration.

The increased potassium secretion induced by a high-potassium intake via the pathways illustrated in Figure 8-3 occurs quite rapidly; moreover, if the intake remains high for more than a few days, a homeostatic phenomenon known as "potassium adaptation" occurs, which is characterized by a marked increase in the ability of the distal nephron to secrete potassium. This adaptation is due mainly to an increase in the actual number of Na-K-ATPase pump sites in the basolateral membrane; aldosterone is at least partly responsible for inducing this change, but other factors may also be involved.

The examples used in this section have been concerned with changes in dietary potassium intake. However, it should be emphasized that when total-body potassium balance is perturbed by primary changes in potassium output, as for example in severe diarrhea, the same mechanisms described above operate homeostatically to control distal potassium secretion and thereby help to restore potassium balance. Thus, the potassium depletion resulting from diarrhea would tend to inhibit aldosterone secretion and, hence, distal potassium secretion.

The phrase "tend to" in the last sentence highlights the fact that, as we have seen, potassium is not the only regulator of aldosterone secretion. The two major controls and the effects of this hormone on sodium and potassium secretion are summarized in Fig. 8-4. (Its third major tubular effect — stimulation of hydrogen-ion secretion — will be described in Chap. 9.) It should be evident that a conflict will arise if decreases (or increases) in *both* potassium and extracellular volume occur simultaneously, since these two changes drive aldosterone production in opposite directions. This is the case in the example of diarrhea.

OTHER FACTORS INFLUENCING POTASSIUM SECRETION

We have now described the mechanisms by which potassium secretion is controlled so as to achieve potassium homeostasis. However, the fact is that potassium secretion is also influenced by factors *not* designed to maintain body potassium constant; indeed, these factors may be so potent as to upset potassium balance. The most important of them clinically are acid-base

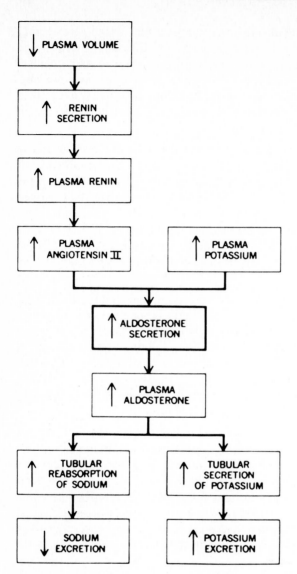

Figure 8-4 Summary of the control of aldosterone and its effects on renal handling of sodium and potassium. Aldosterone exerts a variety of other effects, both renal and nonrenal. Its action on tubular hydrogen-ion secretion is described in Chap. 9. *(From A. J. Vander et al., Human Physiology, © 1970 by McGraw-Hill, Inc. Used with permission of McGraw-Hill Book Company.)*

disturbances and altered renal sodium handling[8] (particularly that due to diuretic drugs). This is because the renal mechanisms for potassium are intimately related to those for sodium and hydrogen ion. The empirical finding that any given factor influences potassium excretion is usually quite straightforward; in contrast, the *mechanism* by which it does so is often much less clear. One should not lose the forest (the empirical finding) for the trees (the likely mechanisms) in these subsequent descriptions. It is very likely that multiple mechanisms are involved in the overall action of each factor, but for simplicity only those considered most important are presented.

Acid-Base Changes

The empirical finding is as follows: The existence of an alkalosis, either metabolic or respiratory in origin, induces increased potassium secretion and excretion (Fig. 8-5). Thus, a primary disturbance in a person's acid-base status can result in a secondary disturbance in potassium balance. For example, a patient suffering from metabolic alkalosis (induced, say, by vomiting) will manifest increased urinary excretion of potassium solely as a result of the alkalosis and will, therefore, become potassium-deficient. (Of course, as soon as potassium balance is upset by these events, the homeostatic mechanisms described in the previous section—for example, decreased aldosterone secretion—will be triggered so as to limit the imbalance.)

The stimulatory effects of alkalosis on potassium secretion appear to be mediated, at least in part, through an increase in the potassium concentration of distal-tubular cells. (This same type of effect of alkalosis on nonrenal-cell potassium concentration was described earlier in this chapter.) It is likely that the presence of an alkalosis somehow stimulates the basolateral potassium-entry step.[9]

What about the presence of an acidosis—does it do just the opposite, i.e., reduce potassium secretion and, thereby, cause potassium retention? For respiratory acidosis and certain forms of metabolic acidosis, the answer is yes, but only during the most acute stages (usually less than 24 h). In other forms of metabolic acidosis there may not even be an acute retention phase because some factor other than the acidosis per

[8] The relationship between the renal handling of sodium chloride and potassium is not a one-way street. Primary changes in potassium balance may have important effects on sodium reabsorption by multiple mechanisms. The text describes one of the indirect influences resulting from potassium-induced changes in aldosterone. There are others, including direct effects of potassium both on tubular sodium reabsorption and on renin secretion. (See Laragh and Sealey, 1973, in Suggested Readings for Chap. 7.)

[9] In addition to this stimulation of distal potassium secretion, distal potassium reabsorption may be inhibited in the presence of an alkalosis. It seems that distal potassium reabsorption requires co-transport with chloride, and distal intraluminal chloride is very low in alkalosis (see Chap. 9).

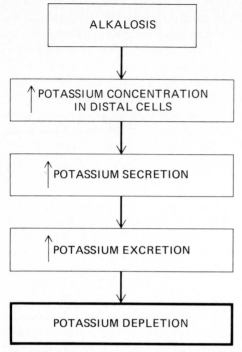

Figure 8-5 Pathway by which alkalosis causes potassium depletion.

se (see below) is enhancing potassium excretion. But the really surprising fact is that even respiratory acidosis and those forms of metabolic acidosis that manifest acute reductions in potassium excretion usually come ultimately to manifest *increased* potassium secretion. Attempts have been made to explain these phenomena,[10] but at the moment the mechanisms by which chronic acidosis alters renal potassium handling remain unclear.

Finally, it should be emphasized that the relationships described here are only one side of the coin; we shall describe in the next chapter how primary changes in potassium balance induce secondary changes in the renal handling of hydrogen ions.

Altered Renal Sodium Handling

The empirical finding is as follows: Potassium excretion is almost always found to be increased when urinary sodium excretion is increased in the following situations: a diet very high in sodium chloride, saline infusion, osmotic diuresis, or diuretic drugs which act on the proximal tubule and/or loop of Henle (Fig. 8-6). The increased potassium excretion is due mainly

[10] See Gennari and Cohen, 1975, in Suggested Readings for Chap. 8.

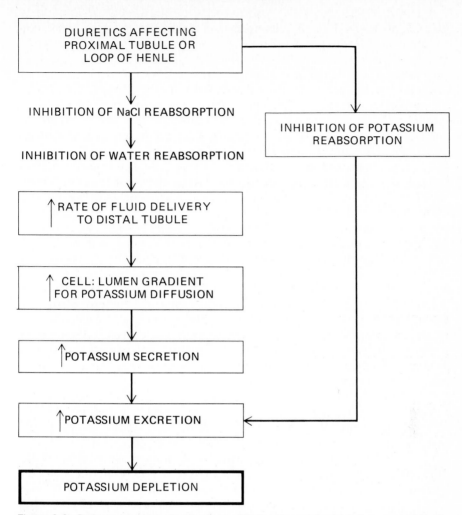

Figure 8-6 Pathway by which diuretic drugs affecting the proximal tubule or loop of Henle cause potassium depletion. The decrease in potassium reabsorption is a less important factor than increased secretion.

to enhanced distal-tubular *secretion*, although as mentioned earlier in this chapter, inhibition of proximal or loop *reabsorption* also makes some contribution to increased *excretion* in all of these situations. Particularly in the last two categories (osmotic diuresis and diuretic drugs), the potassium loss may be severe enough to cause serious potassium depletion.

What is the mechanism for this increased potassium secretion? In all these situations, the volume of fluid flowing into and through the distal tubule per unit time is increased, largely because of inhibition of sodium (or chloride) reabsorption in nephron segments proximal to the distal tubule (see Chaps. 6 and 7). It is this increase in fluid delivery to the potassium-secreting sites in the distal tubule which brings about increased potassium secretion, mainly through the following mechanism. Recall that the final step in potassium secretion — movement across the luminal membrane — is a passive process driven by the concentration gradient for potassium from cell to lumen. Because a large volume flow through the tubule (just by its diluting effect) prevents the luminal concentration from rising rapidly as potassium enters from the cell, the gradient for passive entry is maintained at a high value, and so luminal entry is enhanced.

It should be noted that in the situations listed, the increased volume flow through the distal nephron is due to increased delivery of fluid from more proximal segments. One might have predicted that water diuresis, induced by an absence of ADH, should also cause excretion of large amounts of potassium, since it, too, causes increased fluid flow through the more distal nephron segments, but such is not the case. A major reason is that much of the effect of ADH is distal to the major flow-dependent potassium-secreting sites.

What about situations in which fluid delivery to the distal tubule is significantly *reduced* because of decreased GFR and/or enhanced sodium chloride reabsorption by the proximal tubule or loop? Because of the low volume of fluid, the secretory movement into the lumen of even relatively small amounts of potassium causes the intraluminal concentration to reach a value high enough to abolish the electrochemical gradient for further entry completely; accordingly, a decreased fluid delivery to the distal tubule *tends* to inhibit potassium secretion.[11]

Yet despite this tendency in the two major types of situations that cause distal fluid delivery to be reduced — salt depletion and the diseases of secondary hyperaldosteronism with edema (see Chap. 7) — potassium secretion may be relatively unchanged rather than decreased. The reason for this is that in all these situations plasma aldosterone is elevated (as described in Chap. 7), and the stimulatory effect of aldosterone on potassium secretion counterbalances the inhibitory effect of the reduced fluid delivery to the distal tubule. The net result is that such patients generally manifest relatively normal rates of potassium secretion and excretion. Contrast this to the patient with primary hyperaldosteronism; this person has both an elevated aldosterone and a normal or increased delivery of fluid to the distal tubule (review the changes in renal sodium handling that occur in primary hyperaldosteronism — Chap. 7) and so suffers a marked and persistent elevation in potassium secretion and excretion, enough to cause serious potassium depletion.

Study questions: 60 to 63

---

[11] There is at least one other reason that low flows diminish the electrochemical gradient for potassium movement into the lumen; sodium concentration becomes very low in such situations and this causes the luminal membrane to become more polarized (cell more negative than usual relative to lumen).

CHAPTER 9

RENAL REGULATION OF HYDROGEN-ION BALANCE

OBJECTIVES

The student describes the sources of hydrogen-ion gain and loss; states the major body buffer systems; writes the Henderson-Hasselbalch equation for the CO_2-bicarbonate buffer system and states in general terms the regulation of the two components of this system.

The student understands the renal regulation of extracellular pH.

1 States the role of the kidneys in the regulation of extracellular pH
2 States the two ways in which the kidneys perform this role
3 Calculates the mass of bicarbonate filtered each day
4 Describes the acidifying effect of renal bicarbonate loss
5 Describes the mechanism by which tubular bicarbonate reabsorption occurs; states the role of carbonic anhydrase; quantifies the contributions of the proximal and distal nephron segments to bicarbonate reabsorption
6 Describes how tubular acid secretion can add new bicarbonate to the blood, i.e., lead to the excretion of hydrogen ion
7 States the limiting urine pH, the reason for it, and its significance
8 Defines titratable acid and describes how the measurement is made; states the major buffer(s) which contributes to the formation of titratable acid and its quantitative contributions
9 Describes the role of ammonia in the contribution of new bicarbonate to the blood; defines diffusion trapping and describes how it explains the

relationship between urine pH and ammonium excretion; defines ammonia adaptation to chronic acidosis

10 Distinguishes the rates of acid secretion and excretion; states changes in pH in proximal and distal nephron

11 Calculates, given data, the rate of total acid secretion

12 Calculates, given data, the rate at which the kidneys contribute new bicarbonate to the blood (acid excretion)

13 Describes glomerulotubular balance for bicarbonate

14 Describes the relationship between P_{CO_2} and tubular acid secretion

15 Lists the changes (increase or decrease) of acid secretion, titratable acid excretion, bicarbonate excretion, ammonium excretion, renal addition of new bicarbonate to the blood, and plasma bicarbonate in: metabolic acidosis, metabolic alkalosis, respiratory acidosis, respiratory alkalosis

16 Describes the influence of salt depletion on bicarbonate reabsorption and the capacity of the kidneys to repair an alkalosis; ascribes a specific role to chloride

17 States the effect of increased aldosterone alone on hydrogen-ion secretion

18 States the effect of severe potassium depletion alone on hydrogen-ion secretion

19 Describes how a combination of aldosterone excess and potassium depletion generates a metabolic alkalosis

20 States the effects of large amounts of cortisol or parathyroid hormone on hydrogen-ion secretion

21 Describes how primary changes in acid secretion can influence sodium and chloride reabsorption

22 Describes the urine findings in a patient treated with a carbonic anhydrase inhibitor and the mechanisms responsible

The regulation of total-body hydrogen-ion balance can be viewed in the same way as the balance of any other ion—as the matching of gains and losses. The gastrointestinal absorption of ingested acids or bases contributes to this balance, but this is usually a minor factor (except in individuals who deliberately ingest large quantities of bicarbonate or some other acid or base). Normally, the major route for gain is the metabolic generation of hydrogen ions within the body.

A huge quantity of CO_2 (15,000 to 20,000 mmols) is generated daily as the result of oxidative metabolism and yields hydrogen ions via the reaction:

$$CO_2 + H_2O \rightleftharpoons H_2CO_3 \rightleftharpoons HCO_3^- \text{ and } H^+$$

But this source does not normally constitute a net gain of hydrogen ions, since all those generated via these reactions during passage of blood through the tissues are reincorporated into water when the reactions are reversed during passage of blood through the lungs. Of course, net retention or net elimination of CO_2 (as in hypoventilation or hyperventilation) will result in at least transient gain or loss, respectively, of hydrogen ions.

Another source of metabolic gain of hydrogen ion is the net production of *nonvolatile* or *fixed acids* (so-called to distinguish them from CO_2). These acids include phosphoric and sulfuric (generated during the catabolism of proteins and other organic molecules containing sulfur and phosphorus), lactic acid, ketone bodies, and others. In the United States and most other industrialized countries where the diet is high in protein, people normally have a net daily production of 40 to 80 mmols of these inorganic and organic acids. In contrast, in people whose diet is mainly vegetarian, there is a net metabolic production of alkali rather than hydrogen ions; i.e., the nonvolatile metabolic contribution is actually one of net loss of hydrogen ions.

The third source of net bodily gain or loss of hydrogen ion is the gastrointestinal secretions leaving the body. Vomitus contains a high concentration of hydrogen ions and so constitutes a source of net loss. In contrast, the other gastrointestinal secretions are alkaline, i.e., contain a higher concentration of bicarbonate than exists in plasma, and loss of these fluids (as in diarrhea) constitutes, in essence, a bodily gain of hydrogen ions. This concept, that the excretion of a bicarbonate ion from the body has virtually the same net result as gaining a hydrogen ion, will be developed later in more detail.

Finally, the urine constitutes the fourth source of net hydrogen ion gain or loss. As is the case for the other inorganic ions described in this book, the renal excretion of hydrogen ion is regulated so as to achieve a stable balance and, hence, maintain a relatively stable hydrogen-ion concentration of the body fluids. Thus, the kidneys normally excrete the 40 to 80 mmols of hydrogen ion generated by the average American diet; in contrast, they excrete the required amount of alkali (bicarbonate) in a person whose metabolism is generating net alkali rather than net hydrogen ion. The kidneys also adjust their excretion of hydrogen ion (and bicarbonate) to compensate for any net retention or elimination of CO_2, for any increase in the metabolic production of hydrogen ions (as in diabetic ketoacidosis, for example), and for any increased loss of hydrogen ion or bicarbonate via the gastrointestinal tract.

The idea that hydrogen-ion regulation involves the same kind of input-output balancing as does that of sodium and other ions is easily obscured by the phenomenon of buffering. Thus, between their generation and their elimination, most hydrogen ions are buffered by extracellular and intracellular buffers; i.e., they seem to disappear in a way that sodium ions do not. This buffering is essential for preventing large rises or falls in the hydrogen-ion concentration of the body fluids. For example, the normal extracellular-fluid pH of 7.4 corresponds to an actual hydrogen-ion concentration of only 40 nanomol/L; without buffering interposed between generation and excretion, the daily turnover rate of only the nonvolatile acids—amounting to many millimols (one millimol = one million nanomols) —would cause large changes in pH.

The only important extracellular buffer is the CO_2-HCO_3^- system.

$$H_2O + CO_2 \rightleftharpoons H_2CO_3 \rightleftharpoons H^+ + HCO_3^-$$

The major intracellular buffers are phosphates and proteins. Because all these buffer systems are in equilibrium with each other, a change in one buffer pair will be associated with changes in the others. Accordingly, even though the intracellular buffers account for 50 to 90 percent of the buffering of excess hydrogen ions (depending upon the source of the hydrogen ions), the emphasis in describing the overall regulation of the pH of the body fluids is, for a variety of reasons, generally on the CO_2-HCO_3^- system.

The most important reason for doing so is that there are extremely precise physiological mechanisms for regulating the two critical components of the carbon dioxide–bicarbonate system; the P_{CO_2} is regulated by the respiratory system, and the plasma bicarbonate concentration by the kidneys. As should be evident from the Henderson-Hasselbalch form of the equation, regulation of the P_{CO_2} and bicarbonate concentration achieves regulation of the pH:

$$pH = 6.1 + \log \frac{HCO_3^-}{0.03 \, P_{CO_2}}$$

The kidneys perform their function in two major ways: (1) variable reabsorption of the bicarbonate filtered at the glomerulus, and (2) addition of *new* bicarbonate to the plasma flowing through the kidneys. As we shall see, these two processes are totally interrelated and are, in fact, accomplished by a single mechanism — tubular secretion of hydrogen ion. Inspection of the carbon dioxide–bicarbonate equation above makes it obvious how control of these two renal processes helps to homeostatically regulate extracellular-fluid hydrogen-ion concentration. When plasma hydrogen-ion concentration has been reduced (alkalosis), it can be raised back toward normal by lowering plasma bicarbonate concentration, thereby driving the reaction to the right and generating more hydrogen ion. This the kidneys do by failing to reabsorb all the filtered bicarbonate during alkalosis, allowing this unreabsorbed bicarbonate to be excreted in the urine. *In essence, the excretion of a bicarbonate ion in the urine has virtually the same effect on the blood as would adding a hydrogen ion to the blood.* In contrast to this renal compensation for alkalosis, when plasma hydrogen-ion concentration has been increased (acidosis), the kidneys reabsorb all the filtered bicarbonate and, in addition, contribute new bicarbonate ions (produced by the renal tubular cells) to the blood, thereby shifting the reaction to the left and returning plasma pH toward normal. As we shall see, the renal addition of new bicarbonate to the blood is associated with the excretion of an equal amount of acid in the urine; "the kidney has added new bicarbonate to the blood" and "the kidney has *excreted* acid" are synonymous statements. (Throughout this section the reader must be careful to distinguish between *secretion* and *excretion.*) Thus, to compensate for acidosis, the kidneys excrete an acid urine and alkalinize the blood; in response to alkalosis, they excrete an alkaline urine and acidify the blood.

BICARBONATE REABSORPTION

Bicarbonate is completely filterable at the glomerulus. How much is normally filtered per day?

$$\text{Filtered HCO}_3^-/\text{day} = \text{GFR} \times P_{\text{HCO}_3^-}$$
$$= 180 \text{ L/day} \times 24 \text{ meq/L}$$
$$= 4320 \text{ meq/day}$$

Zero reabsorption of this bicarbonate would be tantamount to adding more than 4 L of 1 N acid to the body. In a normal person virtually all is reabsorbed. Thus, the reabsorption of bicarbonate is normally a conservation process, and essentially none appears in the urine.

How is bicarbonate reabsorbed? One might naturally assume that reabsorption of bicarbonate occurs passively as a result of the same forces described earlier for chloride, but such is the case only for a very small fraction of total bicarbonate reabsorption. There are two reasons for the relative insignificance of passive bicarbonate reabsorption: First, the combined permeability of the luminal-basolateral membranes and/or tight junctions to bicarbonate is relatively low compared to that for chloride. Second, the active-transport process for bicarbonate is so dominant that it greatly reduces any electrochemical gradient favoring net passive movement out of the lumen. (For example, it lowers luminal concentration of bicarbonate.) We will, therefore, ignore any contribution of passive bicarbonate reabsorption across the tubule from lumen to interstitium.

The active reabsorption of bicarbonate is not accomplished in the conventional manner of simply having an active pump for bicarbonate ions at either the luminal or basolateral membrane.[1] Rather, the mechanism by which bicarbonate is reabsorbed involves the secretion of hydrogen ions.

---

[1] This statement is not universally accepted. Some investigators have argued that as much as 40 percent of bicarbonate reabsorption is mediated by an active pump acting upon the bicarbonate ion itself (see Maren, 1974, in Suggested Readings), but the weight of evidence supports the view that such is not the case (see Malnic and Steinmetz, 1976, in Suggested Readings).

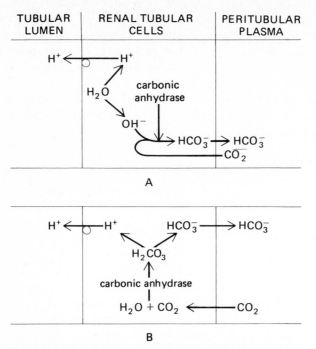

Figure 9-1 Two views of the mechanism of hydrogen-ion secretion. In both: (1) a hydrogen ion is formed in the cell and secreted into the lumen; (2) a bicarbonate ion enters the peritubular plasma from the cell; (3) carbonic anhydrase catalyzes an essential reaction.

Let us look first at the basic process of hydrogen-ion secretion and then apply it to bicarbonate reabsorption.

As shown in Fig. 9-1a, within tubular cells a hydrogen ion and a hydroxyl ion are generated from water; the hydrogen ion is actively secreted into the tubular lumen, leaving the hydroxyl ion behind. This hydroxyl ion combines with CO_2 to form bicarbonate, in a reaction catalyzed by carbonic anhydrase. The bicarbonate ion moves across the basolateral membrane into the interstitial fluid (and then, into the blood) perhaps by facilitated diffusion down its electrochemical gradient (recall that the cell interior is markedly negative relative to the interstitial fluid) or perhaps as a result of some more complicated chemical reaction with enzymes in the membrane. The net result is that for every hydrogen ion secreted into the lumen, a bicarbonate ion enters the blood in the peritubular capillaries.

Although the pathway illustrated in Fig. 9-1a is very likely correct, we will use in subsequent figures the more traditional pathway shown in Fig. 9-1b. In this schema, the hydrogen ion to be secreted is generated from H_2CO_3, and the role of carbonic anhydrase is to catalyze the formation of H_2CO_3 from H_2O and CO_2. We have chosen to use this schema because it is easier to visualize, and it retains a more familiar role for carbonic anhydrase.

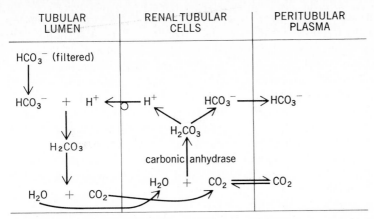

| TUBULAR LUMEN | RENAL TUBULAR CELLS | PERITUBULAR PLASMA |

Figure 9-2 General mechanism by which filtered bicarbonate is reabsorbed. In studying this figure, begin with the carbon dioxide entering the cell from the peritubular plasma. Not shown in the figure are two facts that apply only to the proximal tubule: (1) The breakdown of H_2CO_3 to CO_2 and H_2O in the lumen is also catalyzed by carbonic anhydrase, which is present in the luminal membrane; (2) most of the hydrogen ion is secreted into the lumen via countertransport with sodium.

The mechanism of the active luminal secretory step for hydrogen ions varies in different nephron segments. In the proximal tubule, it is largely via countertransport with sodium entering the cell; i.e., hydrogen-ion secretion in the proximal tubule is largely a secondary active-transport process (see Chap. 2). In contrast, in the distal nephron segments that secrete hydrogen ions (see below), the luminal step probably occurs mainly via a primary hydrogen-ion ATPase pump.

Figure 9-2 illustrates how the overall process of hydrogen-ion secretion achieves bicarbonate reabsorption. Once in the tubular lumen, the secreted hydrogen ion combines with a filtered bicarbonate ion to form carbonic acid; this decomposes to water and carbon dioxide, which diffuse into the cell and then either diffuse into the peritubular plasma or are used by the cell to generate another hydrogen ion and bicarbonate ion. It may seem inaccurate to refer to this process as bicarbonate "reabsorption," since the bicarbonate that appears in the peritubular plasma is not the same bicarbonate ion that was filtered. Yet the overall result is, in effect, the same as it would be if the filtered bicarbonate had been more conventionally reabsorbed like a sodium or potassium ion.

It is also important to note that the hydrogen ion that was *secreted* into the lumen is *not excreted* in the urine. It has been incorporated into water and reabsorbed. The key point here is that any secreted acid (hydrogen ion) that combines with bicarbonate in the lumen to effect bicarbonate reabsorption does not contribute to the urinary *excretion* of acid.

The process of hydrogen-ion secretion and bicarbonate reabsorption occurs throughout the nephron with the exception of the descending loop of Henle. Quantitatively, the proximal tubule is most important in that it reabsorbs approximately 80 to 90 percent of the filtered bicarbonate. The remaining bicarbonate is normally reabsorbed by the ascending loop of Henle, distal tubule, and collecting duct. Throughout the tubule, as shown in Fig. 9-1, *intracellular* carbonic anhydrase is involved in the reactions generating hydrogen ion and bicarbonate. In the proximal tubule, carbonic anhydrase is also located in the luminal cell membranes, and this carbonic anhydrase catalyzes the *intraluminal* decomposition of the very large quantities of carbonic acid formed in this nephron segment. The distal nephron segments do not have luminal-membrane carbonic anhydrase.[2]

ADDITION OF NEW BICARBONATE TO THE PLASMA (RENAL EXCRETION OF ACID)

Besides being able to conserve all the filtered bicarbonate, the kidneys can also contribute *new* bicarbonate to the plasma, so that the mass of bicarbonate in the renal veins exceeds that which entered the kidneys originally. The effect of adding new base to the body is, of course, to alkalinize it, and this is the renal compensation for acidosis.

The mechanism by which new bicarbonate is added to the blood is fundamentally the same as that for bicarbonate reabsorption, namely, tubular acid secretion (Fig. 9-3). The only difference between these two processes is the fate of the secreted hydrogen ions within the tubular lumen. In the case of bicarbonate reabsorption, as we have seen, the secreted acid combines with filtered bicarbonate and is reabsorbed as water; in contrast, in the case of new bicarbonate addition to the blood, the secreted acid combines with other buffers in the lumen (or, to an extremely small degree, remains free in solution) and is excreted. Let us first consider the case in which the secreted acid combines with phosphate, one of the two most important urinary buffers, the other being ammonia.

Note (Fig. 9-3) that the process of hydrogen-ion secretion is the same tubular mechanism described previously, but the net overall effect is different simply because the secreted acid reacts with filtered phosphate rather than with filtered bicarbonate. Therefore, the bicarbonate generated within the tubular cell and entering the plasma constitutes a *net gain* of bicarbonate by the blood, not merely a replacement for a filtered bicarbonate. Thus, when

---

[2] Because of this absence, the intraluminal dissociation of H_2CO_3 to H_2O and CO_2 occurs relatively slowly in these segments, with much of the CO_2 resulting from the dissociation after the urine has left the nephron, i.e., in the lower urinary tract, where the surface-to-volume relationships are unfavorable for the diffusion of CO_2 out of the lumen. Accordingly, for this reason (and others not mentioned here), the urine P_{CO_2} can be much higher than the arterial P_{CO_2} under certain conditions.

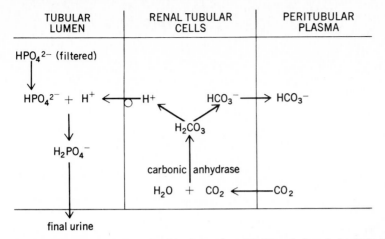

| TUBULAR LUMEN | RENAL TUBULAR CELLS | PERITUBULAR PLASMA |

$HPO_4{}^{2-}$ (filtered)

$HPO_4{}^{2-} + H^+$ ← H^+ $HCO_3{}^-$ → $HCO_3{}^-$

H_2CO_3

$H_2PO_4{}^-$

carbonic anhydrase

$H_2O + CO_2$ ← CO_2

final urine

Figure 9-3 Reaction of secreted hydrogen ion with filtered phosphate. Note that a carbon dioxide molecule has been used up, and a new bicarbonate ion has been released into the blood. In contrast, Fig. 9-2 shows that no net gain or loss of carbon dioxide or bicarbonate occurs when the secreted hydrogen ion is used for bicarbonate reabsorption.

a secreted hydrogen ion combines in the lumen with a buffer other than bicarbonate, the overall effect is not merely one of bicarbonate conservation but rather of addition to the body of *new* bicarbonate, which raises the bicarbonate concentration of the blood and alkalinizes it.

The figure also demonstrates another important point; namely the renal contribution of new bicarbonate to the blood is accompanied by the *excretion* of an equivalent amount of acid in the urine. In this case, in contrast to the reabsorption of bicarbonate, the *secreted* hydrogen ion remains in the tubular fluid, trapped there by the phosphate buffer, and is *excreted* in the urine. This should reinforce the concept that, when the kidneys add new bicarbonate to the blood, they are really excreting hydrogen ion from the body, thereby alkalinizing it. The message should also be clear that the source of essentially all excreted hydrogen ion is tubular secretion. Glomerular filtration of hydrogen ions makes no significant contribution because the concentration of free hydrogen ion at a pH of 7.4, the pH of glomerular filtrate, is less than $10^{-7}M$. Even multiplying this by 180 L/day, one comes up with less than 0.1 mmol filtered per day.

Figure 9-4 illustrates the same process but with ammonia rather than phosphate as the intraluminal buffer. Unlike phosphate, ammonia gains entry to the tubular lumen not by filtration but rather by tubular synthesis and secretion, the mechanism of which will be described later. Again we see that the overall effect is the addition of new bicarbonate to the plasma, combination of the secreted acid with an intraluminal buffer, in this case ammonia, and excretion of the acid.

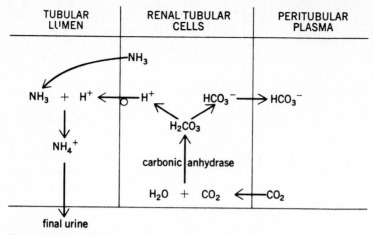

Figure 9-4 Reaction of secreted hydrogen ion with ammonia formed by tubular cells.

The type and quantity of buffers is a crucial determinant of the maximal rate at which the kidneys can excrete acid (contribute new bicarbonate to the blood). This stems from the fact that net addition of hydrogen ions to the lumen ceases when a maximal luminal hydrogen-ion concentration is reached. The reasons for this differ in the proximal and distal nephron. The former, as we have seen, has a relatively leaky epithelium, and, therefore, manifests considerable "pump-leak" characteristics; as the luminal hydrogen-ion concentration rises due to the active entry of hydrogen ions, the gradient for passive diffusion of hydrogen ions from lumen to interstitial fluid increases. Accordingly, a point is reached at which the passive efflux from the lumen exactly equals the active influx from the cells, and no further *net* addition can occur. In contrast, the distal nephron is much less "leaky," and so diffusion out of the lumen is less of a problem. Accordingly, the minimal pH achievable in the distal nephron — 4.4 — is much lower than in the proximal tubule. In fact, back-leakage of hydrogen ions is not the major reason that tubular-fluid pH cannot go below 4.4; the active luminal pump itself is directly inhibited in the presence of a low pH and it virtually ceases to operate when the pH reaches 4.4. Accordingly, the nature and quantity of urinary buffers available to react with the secreted acid and prevent this limiting concentration for free hydrogen ion from being reached is of key importance.

Phosphate and Organic Acids as Buffers

The relationship between monobasic and dibasic phosphate is as follows:

$$HPO_4^{2-} + H^+ \rightleftharpoons H_2PO_4^-$$

This buffer pair provides an excellent buffer system for urine because its pK is 6.8. Expressed in Henderson-Hasselbalch terms:

$$pH = 6.8 + \log\frac{\left[HPO_4^{2-}\right]}{\left[H_2PO_4^-\right]}$$

At the normal pH of plasma and, therefore, of the glomerular filtrate, the equation becomes

$$7.4 = 6.8 + \log\frac{\left[HPO_4^{2-}\right]}{\left[H_2PO_4^-\right]}$$

Solving the equation, we find that there is four times more dibasic $[HPO_4{}^{2-}]$ than monobasic $[H_2PO_4{}^-]$ phosphate in plasma. Therefore, the $HPO_4{}^{2-}$ is available for buffering secreted hydrogen ions. By the time the minimal intratubular pH of 4.4 is reached, virtually all the $HPO_4{}^{2-}$ has been converted to $H_2PO_4{}^-$.

How much $HPO_4{}^{2-}$ is normally filtered per day?[3]

$$\text{Filtered total phosphate/day} = 180 \text{ L/day} \times 1 \text{ mmol/L}$$
$$= 180 \text{ mmol/day}$$
$$\text{Filtered } HPO_4^{2-} = 80\% \times 180 \text{ mmol/day}$$
$$= 144 \text{ mmol/day}$$

However, not all of this filtered $HPO_4{}^{2-}$ is available for buffering, because about 75 percent of filtered phosphate is reabsorbed. Accordingly, unreabsorbed $HPO_4{}^{2-}$ available for buffering is 0.25 × 144 mmol/day = 36 mmol/day. Thus, the reabsorption of phosphate considerably limits the supply of $HPO_4{}^{2-}$ for buffering. Accordingly, as we shall see, ammonia must usually bear the major burden of accepting the additional hydrogen ions in acidosis.

Ammonia and phosphate are normally the only important urinary buffers. However, under abnormal conditions, certain organic buffers may appear in the tubular fluid in large enough quantities to allow them also to act as important buffers. A particularly interesting example is the patient with uncontrolled diabetes mellitus. As a result of insulin deficiency, such a patient may become extremely acidotic because he or she produces large quantities of acetoacetic acid and β-hydroxybutyric acid, which, at plasma pH, almost completely dissociate to yield anions (β-

[3] The number, 1 mM in the equation below, is the value of phosphate in glomerular filtrate; it is somewhat lower than the plasma concentration because a small fraction of plasma phosphate is protein-bound and, therefore, not filterable.

hydroxybutyrate and acetoacetate) and hydrogen ions. These anions are filtered at the glomerulus but are only partly reabsorbed because they are present in great enough quantities to exceed the renal reabsorptive T_ms for them. Accordingly, they are available in the tubular fluid to buffer a portion of the acid being secreted by the tubules to compensate for the acidosis. However, their usefulness in this role is limited by the fact that their pKs are low—approximately 4.5 This means that only about half of these anions will be titrated by secreted acid before the limiting urine pH of 4.4 is reached; i.e., only half of them can actually be used as buffers. If the kidneys could lower the luminal pH to 1, as the stomach can, then it could titrate all of the acetoacetate and β-hydroxybutyrate.

Ammonia as a Buffer

The ammonia-ammonium reaction has a very high pK, approximately 9.2:

$$NH_3 + H^+ \rightleftharpoons NH_4^+$$

$$pH = 9.2 + \log \frac{[NH_3]}{[NH_4^+]}$$

This means that, given the usual urine pH of 7.4 or less, virtually all NH_3 that gains entry to the tubular lumen will immediately pick up hydrogen ions to form NH_4^+. Accordingly, as long as a supply of NH_3 is available, hydrogen-ion secretion and net addition of bicarbonate to the blood can continue with no danger of reaching the minimal urinary pH.

Ammonia Synthesis and Diffusion Trapping

The glomerular filtrate is not a significant source of ammonia because its combined concentration of NH_3-NH_4^+ is very low, and only about 1 percent of even this small amount is in the form of NH_3. (The plasma pH is 7.4 and the reaction pK is 9.2.) Accordingly, the source of ammonia is the renal tubular cells themselves, glutamine serving as the major precursor (Fig. 9-5). The deamidation and deamination of glutamine and its metabolites to yield ammonia proceeds by a variety of metabolic pathways, some in the cytosol and others in the mitochondria, but the single most important one seems to be the two-step reaction mediated by mitochondrial glutaminase and glutamic acid dehydrogenase.[4]

---

[4] In this pathway, the conversion of a molecule of glutamine to α-ketoglutarate generates two hydrogen ions as well as ammonia. However, these two hydrogen ions are eliminated by metabolism of the α-ketoglutarate to glucose (recall that renal tubular cells are capable of gluconeogenesis) or by its complete oxidation to CO_2 and water. Therefore, the renal synthesis of ammonia does not, itself, contribute hydrogen ions to the body.

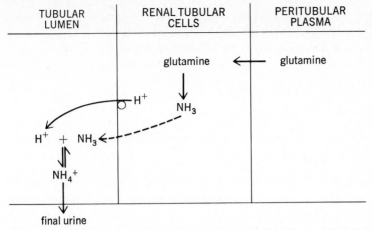

Figure 9-5 Ammonia synthesis and entry into the tubular lumen. (See text for pathways leading to synthesis of ammonia.)

When an individual is acidotic for more than a few days, there occurs a marked increase in ammonia synthesis. This phenomenon, known as *adaptation of ammonia synthesis,* involves enhanced transport of glutamine into mitochondria and/or increased activity of glutaminase. The result of this adaptation (the signal for which is unknown) is that the increased ammonia synthesis provides more ammonia to act as intraluminal buffer, so the kidneys can compensate for the chronic acidosis by contributing a larger amount of new bicarbonate to the blood.

The mechanism by which ammonia, once having been synthesized within the cell, gains entry to the lumen is of considerable importance (Fig. 9-5). It is known as *nonionic diffusion,* or *diffusion trapping,* and its underlying principles were previously described in Chap. 4 in the context of tubular handling of organic solutes. Recall that the ability of a substance to penetrate any cell membrane passively depends upon the lipid solubility of the substance. Accordingly, ammonia, being nonionized, is highly lipid-soluble, whereas ammonium, being charged, is highly lipid-insoluble. Thus, ammonia readily diffuses across renal plasma membranes, whereas ammonium does not. The synthesis of ammonia within the cell creates a cell-lumen concentration gradient down which ammonia diffuses. (Obviously, ammonia will diffuse into the blood also, but we ignore this for the sake of simplicity.) In both the cell and lumen, there exists an equilibrium between ammonia and ammonium. The key point is that the relative amounts of each member of this buffer pair present in the cell and lumen depend upon pH. When the tubular fluid is acid, what happens to the ammonia after it diffuses into the lumen? Immediately, almost all of the ammonia combines with hydrogen ion to form ammonium. Thus, the ammonium concentration in the lumen increases, but since the membrane is virtually impermeable to ammonium, it is trapped within the lumen. Since the ammonia is converted to ammonium almost as fast as it enters, the concentration of ammonia in the lumen is kept low, and the concentration gradient from cell to lumen is maintained. (This assumes that ammonia synthesis keeps pace with exit so as to maintain the intracellular concentration.)

Thus, ammonia passively diffuses into the lumen and is trapped there by conversion to ammonium. The lower the pH of the tubular fluid, the more effective this process, and the more ammonia that enters the lumen. It should be clear, therefore, that this process forces an efficient coupling between renal-tubular acid secretion and the supply of buffer (ammonia) required to react with the secreted hydrogen ion. As the pH of the tubular fluid decreases because of increased acid secretion, the falling pH automatically induces increased entry and trapping of ammonia in the lumen, with subsequent buffering of the hydrogen ions. As long as ammonia synthesis by the cells can keep up with "demand" (unbuffered hydrogen ions in the lumen), then hydrogen-ion secretion can continue without causing the tubular pH to reach the minimal limiting value. The fact that more ammonia synthesis occurs during chronic acidosis (the adaptation process described above) permits ammonia to serve as the major urinary buffer in the kidneys' compensation for acidosis. Ammonium excretion may increase from a normal value of 20 meq/day to 500 meq/day in a person suffering from severe acidosis. In contrast, phosphate's contribution may increase by only 20 to 40 meq/day.

The other side of this coin should also be emphasized: When the urine is not acid, there will be little diffusion trapping of ammonia. Unless enough acid is secreted by the tubules to force a significant reduction of tubular-fluid pH, little ammonium will be excreted in the urine.

We have so far said nothing about the sites of ammonia synthesis and entry into the lumen. This substance is produced by both the proximal tubule and distal nephron segments, but since the lowest tubular-fluid pH occurs in the distal nephron, it is here that maximum diffusion trapping occurs.[5]

QUALITATIVE INTEGRATION OF BICARBONATE REABSORPTION AND ACID EXCRETION

To reiterate, acid secreted by the tubules can suffer one of two general fates: (1) It can combine with filtered bicarbonate, in which case the overall process accomplishes bicarbonate reabsorption. (2) Or it can combine with filtered nonbicarbonate buffers (such as phosphate) or with ammonia that has been synthesized and secreted by the tubules.

---

[5] It is likely that, even during acidosis, much of the ammonia entering the collecting ducts was actually synthesized in the proximal tubule and then "short-circuited" from the loop of Henle into the collecting ducts. This process is summarized in Sajo *et al.* (Suggested Readings).

The first case is a conservation process, by which the kidneys prevent loss of bicarbonate from the body. This process alone does not alkalinize the body but rather prevents the development of an acidosis due to bicarbonate loss. In contrast, the second process contributes new bicarbonate to the body and simultaneously excretes acid, thereby alkalinizing it.

What determines whether the secreted hydrogen ions, once in the lumen, combine with bicarbonate, on the one hand, or with phosphate, ammonia, or organic buffers, on the other? This depends upon the pKs of each buffer-pair reaction and upon the mass of each buffer present. To simplify matters, one may assume that, compared to bicarbonate, relatively little nonbicarbonate buffer is titrated, i.e., combines with hydrogen ion, until most of the bicarbonate has been reabsorbed. This is true mainly because the quantity of bicarbonate is huge compared to the quantity of the other buffers. Once most of the filtered bicarbonate has been reabsorbed, then almost all of the secreted acid combines with the other buffers.

This analysis also explains the contributions of the different nephron segments to these processes. The proximal tubule secretes far more hydrogen ion than does the distal nephron, and most of this proximally secreted hydrogen ion goes to achieve bicarbonate reabsorption (90 percent is reabsorbed proximally); the pH of the intratubular fluid falls less than 1 pH unit, and only a small amount of hydrogen ion is picked up by phosphate and other buffers. In contrast, because relatively little bicarbonate normally remains by the beginning of the distal tubule, the hydrogen ions secreted by this nephron segment and the collecting duct can reabsorb it and then create the low pH required both for titration of nonbicarbonate urinary buffers and for the diffusion trapping of ammonia. However, should a large amount of bicarbonate escape proximal reabsorption, then most of the hydrogen ions secreted by the distal nephron segments, too, would be expended in reabsorbing bicarbonate rather than in titrating urinary buffers.

One can imagine, then, a spectrum of events reflecting the acid-base status of the body.

Alkalosis

When an alkalosis exists, the kidneys compensate by secreting too little acid to accomplish complete reabsorption of filtered bicarbonate. Therefore, bicarbonate is excreted in an alkaline urine (pH >7.4), and the body is thereby made more acid. Simultaneously, because the acid secreted is inadequate to reabsorb all the bicarbonate, there is virtually no hydrogen ion available to combine with nonbicarbonate buffers. This is just what one would expect teleologically, since the kidneys are "attempting" to eliminate bicarbonate from the body, not add new bicarbonate to it.

Normal State

Metabolism of the average American diet results in the net liberation, per person, of 40 to 80 meq of hydrogen ion per day. Therefore, if balance is to be maintained, the kidneys must excrete this same amount of acid, i.e., contribute 40 to 80 meq of new bicarbonate to the blood. (Again, we emphasize that these are synonymous statements.) Accordingly, tubular acid secretion must be great enough to effect complete reabsorption of all filtered bicarbonate, and an additional 40 to 80 meq acid must be secreted to contribute 40 to 80 meq new bicarbonate to the blood, this acid being excreted in the urine buffered by phosphate and ammonia. The urine under such circumstances is moderately acid, perhaps at pH 6.

Acidosis

The kidneys compensate for acidosis by adding large quantities of new bicarbonate to the blood. Therefore, as in the previously described normal state, acid secretion must be great enough to effect complete reabsorption of all filtered bicarbonate. Beyond this, the tubules must secrete large amounts of additional acid so as to add an equivalent amount of new bicarbonate to the blood. This acid is excreted in the urine buffered by phosphate and ammonia (and by organic buffers, when they are present). Under such conditions, ammonia usually becomes the most important buffer; its supply by diffusion trapping is assured by the fact that once all the bicarbonate is reabsorbed, the large continued secretion of acid causes the tubular-fluid pH to fall progressively toward the minimal pH of 4.4.

It should now be clear how, via changes in the rate of a single variable, namely, the rate of tubular acid secretion, the kidneys can compensate for the entire range of acid-base patterns that can occur. The factors that regulate this process in response to acid-base changes will be discussed after the following section detailing the methods for *quantitating* renal handling of hydrogen ion.

QUANTITATION OF RENAL ACID-BASE FUNCTIONS

Measurement of Tubular Acid-Secretion Rate

A hydrogen ion secreted by the tubules can combine in the lumen with bicarbonate, phosphate, ammonia, or one of several organic buffers. In order to calculate the total mass of acid secreted per unit time, one must add up the contributions of all these pathways. The amount of free hydrogen ion may be ignored because it is so small.

It is worthwhile to emphasize once more the great difference between the fate of a hydrogen ion reacting with bicarbonate and the fate of one reacting with any of the other buffers. As described above, the combination of a hydrogen ion with bicarbonate causes the generation of carbon dioxide and water, both of which are reabsorbed by the tubules. Thus, the secreted hydrogen ion that is used for bicarbonate reabsorption does not remain in the urine. How, then, can one measure it? The answer reflects the fact that one bicarbonate ion is reabsorbed as a result of the secretion of one hydrogen ion. Therefore, assuming this one-to-one ratio, we can calculate the mass of secreted hydrogen ion reacting with bicarbonate by measuring the rate of bicarbonate reabsorption. The rate is equal to the difference between filtered and excreted bicarbonate. For example, given the following data, how much secreted acid combined in the lumen with bicarbonate?

$$\left. \begin{array}{l} \text{GFR} = 180 \text{ L/day} \\ P_{HCO_3^-} = 24 \text{ meq/L} \\ \text{Urine vol} = 1 \text{ L/day} \\ U_{HCO_3^-} = 24 \text{ meq/L} \end{array} \right\} \text{Basic data}$$

$$\begin{aligned} \text{Filtered } HCO_3^-/\text{day} &= \text{GFR} \times P_{HCO_3^-} \\ &= 180 \text{ L/day} \times 24 \text{ meq/L} \\ &= 4320 \text{ meq/day} \end{aligned}$$

$$\begin{aligned} \text{Excreted } HCO_3^-/\text{day} &= U_{HCO_3^-} \times V \\ &= 24 \text{ meq/L} \times 1 \text{ L/day} \\ &= 24 \text{ meq/day} \end{aligned}$$

$$\begin{aligned} \text{Reabsorbed } HCO_3^-/\text{day} &= \text{filtered } HCO_3^-/\text{day} - \text{excreted } HCO_3^-/\text{day} \\ &= 4320 \text{ meq/day} - 24 \text{ meq/day} \\ &= 4296 \text{ meq/day} \end{aligned}$$

Thus, 4296 meq H^+ must have been secreted to accomplish the reabsorption of 4296 meq HCO_3^-.

In contrast to the hydrogen ion that reacts with bicarbonate, the one that combines with phosphate, organic buffers, and ammonia does remain in the tubular fluid and is excreted in the urine bound to these buffers. Except for that which combines with NH_3, this quantity of acid can be measured by taking a sample of urine and titrating it with sodium hydroxide back to pH of 7.4, the pH of the plasma from which the glomerular filtrate originated. This simply reverses the events that occurred within the tubular lumen when the tubular fluid was titrated by secreted hydrogen ions. Thus, the number of milliequivalents of sodium hydroxide required to reach pH 7.4 must equal the number of milliequivalents of hydrogen ion added to the tubular fluid that combined with phosphate and the organic buffers. This value is known as the *titratable acid.*

It must be stressed that the titratable-acid measurement does *not* pick up hydrogen ions that combined with ammonia to yield ammonium. The reason is that the pK of the ammonia-ammonium reaction is so high (9.2) that titration with alkali to pH 7.4 will not remove the hydrogen ions from the ammonium. In addition to measuring titratable acid, therefore, a separate measurement of urinary ammonium excretion must be performed.

The total rate of tubular hydrogen-ion *secretion* is thus equal to the sum of:

HCO_3^- reabsorption meq/time

+ titratable acid, meq/time

+ NH_4^+ excretion, meq/time

Values for a person on a normal diet are approximately:

HCO_3^- reabsorption = 4300 meq/day

Titratable acid = 20 meq/day

NH_4^+ excretion = 40 meq/day

These values serve to emphasize that the vast majority of secreted hydrogen ions are used to accomplish bicarbonate reabsorption, with only a small number remaining for excretion—the production of titratable acid or ammonium.

Measurement of Renal Contribution of New Bicarbonate to the Blood

The above analysis also indicates how to calculate the amount of *new* bicarbonate added to the blood by the kidneys, an extremely important number, since it is a measurement of the degree to which the kidneys have alkalinized the body. It is simply the sum of titratable acid and ammonium. (Again, the amount of free hydrogen ion may be ignored because it is so small.) This sum measures the rate of acid *excreted* in the urine secondary to tubular acid secretion, and, as we have stressed several times, it is identical to the quantity of new bicarbonate added by the renal tubular cells to the blood. This stems from the fact that each hydrogen ion secreted into the lumen that reacts with a nonbicarbonate buffer remains in the tubular fluid and is excreted.

We can now state the data required for a quantitative assessment of the renal contribution to acid-base regulation in any patient:

---

1 Titratable acid excreted

2 + NH_4^+ excreted

3 − HCO_3^- excreted (i.e., filtered HCO_3^- lost from the body because of incomplete reabsorption)

Total = net HCO_3^- gain or loss to the body (negative values equal loss, positive values equal gain).

Typical urine data for the renal compensations in the three states described are as follows:

Alkalosis

$$\begin{aligned}
\text{Titratable acid} &= 0 \text{ meq/day}\\
+ NH_4^+ &= 0 \text{ meq/day}\\
- HCO_3^- \text{ excreted} &= -80 \text{ meq/day}
\end{aligned}$$

80 meq HCO_3^- *lost* from the body

(Urine pH = 8.0)

Normal state

$$\begin{aligned}
\text{Titratable acid} &= 20 \text{ meq/day}\\
+ NH_4^+ &= 40 \text{ meq/day}\\
- HCO_3^- \text{ excreted} &= -1 \text{ meq/day}
\end{aligned}$$

59 meq HCO_3^- *added* to the body

(Urine pH = 6.0)

Acidosis

$$\begin{aligned}
\text{Titratable acid} &= 40 \text{ meq/day}\\
+ NH_4^+ &= 160 \text{ meq/day}\\
- HCO_3^- \text{ excreted} &= 0 \text{ meq/day}
\end{aligned}$$

200 meq HCO_3^- *added* to the body

(Urine pH = 4.6)

It should be emphasized that the data shown for alkalosis are typical of respiratory alkalosis and "pure" metabolic alkalosis, i.e., alkalosis uncomplicated by other electrolyte abnormalities. As we shall see in subsequent sections, electrolyte imbalances frequently complicate the picture in metabolic alkalosis so that the urine may not be alkaline.

HOMEOSTATIC CONTROL OF RENAL TUBULAR ACID SECRETION

There are multiple factors which control the key element in the kidney's acid-base machinery, the rate of tubular hydrogen-ion secretion. Several of these factors control acid secretion so as to homeostatically regulate the pH of the body fluids.

Glomerulotubular Balance for Bicarbonate

One of the important influences on hydrogen-ion secretion is analogous to the phenomenon of glomerulotubular balance previously described for

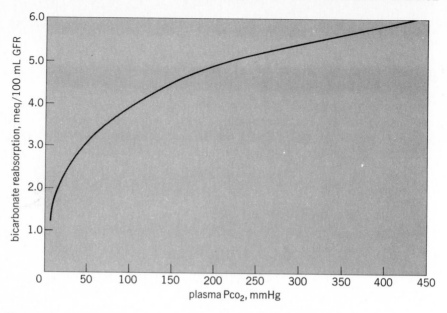

Figure 9-6 The relationship between P_{CO_2} of arterial blood and reabsorption of bicarbonate in the dog. [*Data from F. C. Rector, Jr., et al., J. Clin. Invest.,* **39**:*1706 (1960)*.]

sodium. Hydrogen-ion secretion (and, therefore, bicarbonate reabsorption) varies directly with GFR. For example, if GFR increases 25 percent, so does bicarbonate reabsorption. The adaptive value of such a relationship is that changes in GFR do not induce potentially serious perturbations in the acid-base status of the body. In the example of the 25 percent increase cited above, if acid secretion and bicarbonate reabsorption did not increase proportionally to GFR, a very large quantity of bicarbonate would be lost from the body with a resulting acidosis. The mechanism responsible for bicarbonate glomerulotubular balance very likely is part of the same overall process that achieves glomerulotubular balance for sodium.

P_{CO_2} and Renal Intracellular pH

The most important single determinant of the rate of tubular acid secretion, so far as homeostatic regulation is concerned, is the P_{CO_2} of the arterial blood. As shown in Fig. 9-6, the rate of hydrogen-ion secretion, as manifested by bicarbonate reabsorptive rate, is directly related to the P_{CO_2} of the arterial plasma. (In this figure, bicarbonate reabsorption is expressed in milliequivalents per 100 mL GFR rather than in milliequivalents per time because of the previously described influence of glomerulotubular balance.) This relationship holds over the entire range of arterial P_{CO_2} values.

There are no nerves or hormones mediating this response; rather, the renal tubular cells respond to the P_{CO_2} of the blood perfusing them. An increased P_{CO_2} of arterial blood causes, by diffusion of carbon dioxide, an equivalent increase in P_{CO_2} within the tubular cells. This causes, by mass action, an elevated intracellular hydrogen-ion concentration, and it is presumably this change that directly stimulates the rate of hydrogen-ion secretion. In other words, the ultimate stimulus for hydrogen-ion secretion is not the P_{CO_2} per se but rather the decreased intracellular pH it induces.[6]

The reason that intracellular pH is so responsive to changes in arterial P_{CO_2} is the ease with which carbon dioxide diffuses across cell membranes. Thus, a small change in blood P_{CO_2} causes an almost immediate equivalent change in cell P_{CO_2}, which, by mass action, alters cell pH. In contrast to this sensitivity to P_{CO_2} changes, cell pH is much less dependent upon changes in blood pH per se—the reasons being that cell membranes are less permeable to the diffusion of hydrogen ion itself (or of bicarbonate) and that transport mechanisms for hydrogen ion at the basolateral membrane can minimize the transmission of extracellular pH changes into the cell. This is not to say that the cells are completely impervious to extracellular pH changes unaccompanied by simultaneous changes in P_{CO_2}. Such extracellular pH changes (particularly when chronic) generally do influence intracellular pH but much less than extracellular P_{CO_2} changes do. Accordingly, the rate or renal acid secretion correlates better with blood P_{CO_2} than with blood pH.[7]

Renal Compensation for Respiratory Acidosis and Alkalosis

Let us apply this analysis to two clinical situations, respiratory acidosis and alkalosis. For reference, we shall present the basic equations again. (CO_2 rather than H_2CO_3 can be used in the second equation because their concentrations are always in direct proportion to one another.)

$$H_2O + CO_2 \rightleftharpoons H_2CO_3 \rightleftharpoons H^+ + HCO_3^-$$

$$[H^+] = K\frac{[CO_2]}{[HCO_3^-]}$$

[6] This effect of P_{CO_2} on intracellular pH is not the only way in which P_{CO_2} influences acid secretion. For example, an increased P_{CO_2} stimulates insertion of H^+ pumps in the luminal membrane. Moreover, recent evidence suggests that some of the influence of P_{CO_2} is not exerted directly on the kidney at all but is the indirect consequence of altered cardiovascular function. (See Arruda and Kurtzman, 1978, in Suggested Readings.)

[7] This discussion has been in terms of the influence of intracellular pH on hydrogen-ion secretion. It is possible that the extracellular pH also directly influences hydrogen-ion secretion. (See Suggested Readings.)

In chronic pulmonary insufficiency, carbon dioxide is retained, and the resulting increase in P_{CO_2} drives the carbon dioxide–bicarbonate reaction to the right, with a resulting acidosis. It should be clear from both equations that the pH could be restored to normal if the bicarbonate could be elevated to the same degree as the P_{CO_2}. There is, of course, an automatic increase in bicarbonate concentration solely as a result of the reaction being driven to the right by the elevated P_{CO_2}, but this is not nearly to the same degree as the rise in P_{CO_2}. If we transpose the second equation, we can see why mass action alone does not lead to proportionate increases of bicarbonate and carbon dioxide when P_{CO_2} increases:

$$[H^+][HCO_3^-] \rightleftharpoons K[CO_2]$$

This form of the equation emphasizes that a rise in carbon dioxide causes a proportionate rise in the *product* $[H^+]$ $[HCO_3^-]$. Since hydrogen-ion concentration increases, bicarbonate concentration cannot increase as much as carbon dioxide does or else their product would rise more than proportionally. (Plug in some numbers and convince yourself this is true.)

It is the kidneys' job to cause the additional bicarbonate increase by contributing new bicarbonate to the blood. This occurs because the increased P_{CO_2} stimulates renal-tubular acid secretion so that all filtered bicarbonate is reabsorbed and much secreted acid is left over for the formation of titratable acid and ammonium, i.e., for the addition of new bicarbonate to the blood. This process continues until a new steady state is reached, at which point the plasma bicarbonate is so high that even the enhanced rate of acid secretion can serve only to reabsorb the increased filtered load of bicarbonate $-$ GFR $\times$ P_{HCO_3} $-$ and cannot contribute large amounts of new bicarbonate. The renal compensation is not usually perfect; i.e., when the steady state is reached, the plasma bicarbonate is not elevated to quite the same degree as is the P_{CO_2}. Consequently, blood pH is not completely returned to normal.

The sequence of events in response to respiratory alkalosis is just the opposite. Respiratory alkalosis is the result of hyperventilation, in which the patient transiently eliminates carbon dioxide faster than it is produced, thereby lowering his or her P_{CO_2} and raising pH. The decreased P_{CO_2} reduces tubular acid secretion so that bicarbonate reabsorption is not complete. Bicarbonate is then lost from the body, and the loss results in a decreased plasma bicarbonate and a return toward normal plasma pH.

Renal Compensation for Metabolic Acidosis and Alkalosis

The primary cause of so-called metabolic acidosis is either the addition to the body (by ingestion, infusion, or production) of increased amounts of an acid other than carbonic acid, or alternatively, the loss from the body of bicarbonate (as in diarrhea). Inspection of the equations reveals that either loss of bicarbonate or addition of hydrogen ions will lower both the plasma pH and the plasma bicarbonate concentration. The kidney compensation is to raise the plasma bicarbonate concentration back toward normal, thereby returning pH toward normal. In order to do this, the kidneys must reabsorb all the filtered bicarbonate and contribute new bicarbonate through the formation of titratable acid and ammonium. This is precisely what normal kidneys do, and the urines excreted in respiratory and metabolic acidosis are indistinguishable in these respects.

Yet the surprising fact is that in metabolic acidosis (in contrast to respiratory acidosis), these events occur in the absence of a significant stimulus to the kidney to increase acid secretion; indeed, they frequently occur in the presence of a decreased stimulus, since the PCO_2 of arterial blood, which is the major stimulus for tubular acid secretion, as described above, is *not increased* in metabolic acidosis but is usually *decreased*. Why? Because, as the arterial pH falls as a result of whatever is causing the metabolic acidosis, pulmonary ventilation is reflexly stimulated. This is, of course, the respiratory compensation for the acidosis, and its effect is to reduce arterial PCO_2. Therefore, because renal-tubular-cell pH is rapidly altered by changes in PCO_2, renal-tubular-cell pH is likely to be *increased* in the early stages of metabolic acidosis. (In patients with chronic metabolic acidosis, it is likely that intracellular pH returns to normal or actually decreases, despite a continued decrease in PCO_2, probably because of altered basolateral-membrane transport of hydrogen ion.)

How, then, can the kidneys manage to perform their compensatory function with no stimulus to increase acid secretion? This apparent paradox is resolved when one recalls that in uncompensated metabolic acidosis the plasma bicarbonate is lower than normal. (In contrast, during respiratory acidosis plasma bicarbonate is greater than normal, even in the uncompensated state.) Therefore, the mass of bicarbonate filtered (GFR $\times$ P_{HCO3^-}) is reduced proportionally to the decreased plasma bicarbonate, and less hydrogen ion need be secreted to accomplish its total reabsorption. Accordingly, even with a decreased total acid secretion, there is still considerable hydrogen ion available after the bicarbonate has been completely reabsorbed to form large amounts of titratable acid and ammonium, i.e., to contribute new bicarbonate to the plasma. For example, compare the data for a person with metabolic acidosis with those for a normal person:

		Normal	*Metabolic acidosis*
Plasma HCO_3^-	Basic data	24 meq/L	12 meq/L
GFR		180 L/day	180 L/day
Filtered HCO_3^-		4320 meq/day	2160 meq/day
1 Reabsorbed HCO_3^-		4315 meq/day	2160 meq/day
2 Titratable acid and NH_4^+		60 meq/day	200 meq/day
3 Total H^+ secreted [(1) + (2)]		4375 meq/day	2360 meq/day

Thus, even in the presence of a greatly reduced acid secretion, the kidneys are able to compensate for the metabolic acidosis. Indeed, the limiting factor in this type of acidosis turns out to be not the rate of acid secretion but rather the availability of buffer. For example, in the situation of metabolic acidosis just described, although the ability of the tubules to secrete hydrogen ion may well have been somewhat reduced by the presence of a low P_{CO_2}, they certainly could have secreted more than 2360 meq if more buffer were available. Moreover, recent evidence suggests that the rate of hydrogen-ion secretion by the collecting ducts (in contrast to the distal tubules) may actually be increased during metabolic acidosis, despite the reflexly reduced P_{CO_2}; the mechanism is unknown, but may involve aldosterone (see below).

The situation in metabolic alkalosis is just the opposite. Despite a normal or increased rate of acid secretion (secondary to a reflexly elevated P_{CO_2}) the load of filtered bicarbonate is so great that much bicarbonate escapes reabsorption,[8] and no titratable acid or ammonium can be formed. Therefore, plasma bicarbonate is decreased, and pH decreases toward normal.[9]

OTHER FACTORS INFLUENCING HYDROGEN-ION SECRE-TION

The previous section described the mechanisms by which hydrogen-ion secretion is controlled so as to achieve acid-base homeostasis. We now describe how factors *not* designed to maintain pH constant can also influence hydrogen-ion secretion and bicarbonate reabsorption. In other words, just as is true for potassium, hydrogen-ion balance has its own distinct homeostatic controls, but it is also at the mercy of other interacting factors. The most important of these are aldosterone, extracellular-volume contraction, and potassium depletion. (Again, similarly to the situation for potassium, such interactions are the result of the close interlinking of renal sodium, potassium, chloride, and hydrogen-ion handling.) These factors may have two general effects: First, they may cause the kidneys to generate an acid-base disorder in the body by secreting too much or too little hydrogen ion; second, their presence may not cause the kidneys to generate an acid-base disorder but may prevent them from doing their usual job of compensating for an already existing acid-base disorder.

---

[8] Recent experiments suggest that during metabolic alkalosis, not only does some bicarbonate escape reabsorption, but there may actually occur *secretion* of bicarbonate ions into the collecting ducts. If this proves to be true, the overall picture of renal bicarbonate handling will obviously require reevaluation.

[9] Recent evidence suggests that this description of how the kidney manages to increase bicarbonate excretion despite the stimulus to hydrogen-ion secretion exerted by a reflexly elevated P_{CO_2} may not fully apply to chronic situations. (See Madras *et al.* in Suggested Readings.)

Influence of Salt Depletion on Acid Secretion

The presence of salt depletion and extracellular-volume contraction interferes with the ability of the kidneys to compensate for a metabolic alkalosis. In metabolic alkalosis, the plasma bicarbonate is elevated, either because of addition of bicarbonate to the body or because of loss of acid from it. The normal renal compensation should be to set hydrogen-ion secretion at a level that fails to achieve complete bicarbonate reabsorption and thereby allows the excess bicarbonate to be excreted. But the presence of the salt depletion not only stimulates sodium reabsorption but also stimulates hydrogen-ion secretion. The actual mechanisms by which the salt depletion enhances hydrogen-ion secretion are unclear at present, but the effect is mainly on proximal hydrogen-ion secretion.[10] The net result is that all of the filtered bicarbonate is reabsorbed so that the already elevated plasma bicarbonate associated with the preexisting metabolic alkalosis is locked in, and the plasma pH remains unchanged; instead of being alkaline as it should, the urine is somewhat acid.

It should be emphasized that salt depletion will not usually induce the kidneys to *generate* a metabolic alkalosis; rather, it merely reduces their ability to *compensate* for a metabolic alkalosis once the alkalosis is established from some other cause. The major reason that salt depletion alone does not *cause* an alkalosis is that it usually has relatively little stimulating effect on the distal nephron's generation of titratable acid and ammonium. In other words, salt depletion per se induces complete reabsorption of filtered bicarbonate but little or no renal contribution of new bicarbonate. If the plasma bicarbonate level is normal to start with, reabsorption of all the filtered bicarbonate merely maintains the same normal plasma bicarbonate level. It does not increase plasma bicarbonate level. The situation is analogous to the reabsorption of glucose in normal individuals; i.e., reabsorption of all the filtered glucose merely keeps plasma glucose at the normal level.

Finally, it should be noted that we have referred to salt depletion in this section without distinguishing between sodium and chloride losses. This is because loss of either of these ions will lead to extracellular-volume contraction. There has been considerable controversy concerning a possible additional effect of chloride deficiency: Does specific chloride depletion, in a manner independent of extracellular volume contraction, help maintain metabolic alkalosis by stimulating hydrogen-ion secretion? The answer is probably yes; the mechanisms for the specific chloride-depletion effect remain unclear, but the phenomenon may have considerable clinical importance.

---

[10] A distal-tubular effect can also be revealed with appropriate experimental manipulations but does not make an important contribution in most clinical situations associated with salt depletion.

Aldosterone Excess and Potassium Depletion

This section discusses an excellent example of how two distinct inputs, each relatively small by itself, can together produce a major effect of great clinical significance. First we will consider the individual effects.

Aldosterone (as well as other mineralocorticoids) stimulates hydrogen-ion secretion (and ammonia production) by a direct action on the distal tubules and collecting ducts. This effect seems to be quite distinct from aldosterone's actions on sodium reabsorption and potassium secretion. By itself, this direct effect is relatively small but it does have physiological significance. For one thing, even at its usual plasma concentrations, aldosterone probably tonically facilitates hydrogen-ion secretion. Second, its plasma concentration increases during metabolic acidosis (because increased renin secretion → increased plasma angiotensin II → increased aldosterone secretion), and this may contribute to the increased secretion of hydrogen ion by the collecting ducts seen in this state and mentioned earlier. Finally, increased plasma aldosterone may also contribute to the increased hydrogen-ion secretion observed during salt depletion, although, as described above, other proximally acting factors seem more important in that condition. It must be emphasized that we have thus far been describing only the relatively small tubular effects of aldosterone alone on hydrogen-ion secretion. We shall see that when to this effect is added another event — potassium depletion — then a marked increase in hydrogen-ion secretion is induced.

Potassium depletion, by itself, also tends to stimulate tubular hydrogen-ion secretion (and ammonia production). Presumably, potassium depletion of renal tubular cells causes a decrease in renal-cell pH (because of the reciprocal relations between cell pH and potassium described in the previous chapter), and it is this decrease which stimulates hydrogen-ion secretion. For many years, it has been argued whether potassium depletion, by itself, can stimulate tubular hydrogen-ion secretion enough to significantly alter the renal contribution to acid-base balance. Most evidence now indicates that this may sometimes be the case in people, but only when the degree of potassium depletion is extremely severe.[11]

Now we come to the critical point. The combination of potassium depletion of even moderate degree and high levels of aldosterone acts synergistically to markedly stimulate tubular hydrogen-ion secretion. As a result, the renal tubules not only reabsorb all filtered bicarbonate but contribute inappropriately large amounts of new bicarbonate to the body, thereby *causing* the development of metabolic alkalosis. Note that there

[11] One reason for the failure of potassium depletion by itself to produce a significant excess of hydrogen-ion secretion is that potassium depletion inhibits secretion of aldosterone (as described in Chap. 8). Accordingly, the stimulatory effect aldosterone tonically exerts on hydrogen-ion secretion is lost, and this loss offsets the stimulatory effect exerted by potassium depletion. (See Suggested Readings for Chap. 9.)

may have been nothing wrong with the acid-base balance to start with: The alkalosis is actually generated by the kidneys themselves. (Of course, if alkalosis were already present due to some other cause, the presence of this high-aldosterone–potassium-depletion combination would not only prevent the kidneys from compensating but would make the alkalosis worse.)

This phenomenon is important because the combination of a markedly elevated aldosterone and potassium depletion occurs in a variety of clinical situations. One reason for their coexistence is that the former can cause the latter. Recall from Chap. 8 that aldosterone stimulates potassium secretion; therefore, a very high level of aldosterone may cause potassium depletion via the urine. The potassium depletion and high aldosterone then act together to induce the kidneys to generate an alkalosis. A good example of this is the patient with primary hypersecretion of aldosterone due to an adrenal tumor (Fig. 9-7).

Another common situation in which a high plasma-aldosterone concentration and potassium depletion coexist is the extensive use of diuretic drugs (Fig. 9-8). This combination can then act to generate a metabolic alkalosis. Note also that the person in this example is triply in trouble —as described in the previous section of this chapter, salt depletion per se (via mechanisms unrelated to aldosterone) stimulates reabsorption of bicarbonate and, therefore, helps to maintain the alkalosis once the high-aldosterone–potassium-depletion combination has generated it.

Given the ability of combined aldosterone excess and potassium depletion to generate metabolic alkalosis, one might logically predict that the combination of pathologic aldosterone deficiency and potassium retention (the latter usually due to the former) might induce metabolic acidosis by partially inhibiting renal tubular secretion of hydrogen ion. Such is, in fact, the case, as illustrated by the modest metabolic acidosis manifested by patients with the inability to secrete aldosterone normally.

Cortisol and Parathyroid Hormone

A number of hormones other than aldosterone are capable of influencing tubular hydrogen-ion secretion when they are present in very high concentrations. Of these, the most important clinically are cortisol and parathyroid hormone. Cortisol's actions are quite similar to those of aldosterone and may simply reflect the fact that high concentrations of this hormone, physiologically a glucocorticoid, can exert mineralocorticoid effects: sodium retention, potassium depletion, and metabolic alkalosis.

Parathyroid hormone's major physiological role as regulator of calcium homeostasis will be decribed in the next chapter. Quite distinct from its actions on calcium, parathyroid hormone can inhibit hydrogen-ion secretion by the proximal tubule, resulting in excessive loss of bicarbonate via the urine and the development of a metabolic acidosis. This may be an important influence in patients who have excessive blood concentrations of parathyroid

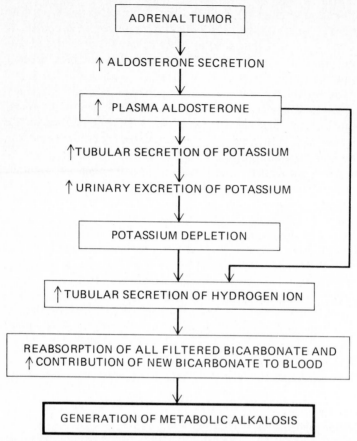

Figure 9-7 Pathway for generation of metabolic alkalosis in a patient with primary hyperaldosteronism. The increased aldosterone is itself the cause of the potassium depletion.

hormone, and some investigators believe that the response occurs at low enough concentrations for it to be a normal physiological regulator of acid-base balance; this latter hypothesis remains to be proven.

INFLUENCE OF HYDROGEN-ION SECRETION ON SODIUM CHLORIDE REABSORPTION

The previous sections described how alterations in salt balance could influence hydrogen-ion secretion. This section deals with the reverse phenomenon, the ability of primary changes in hydrogen-ion secretion and bicarbonate reabsorption to alter sodium and chloride handling.

As mentioned earlier, hydrogen-ion secretion in the proximal tubule is directly coupled to the countertransport of sodium; i.e., sodium is literally

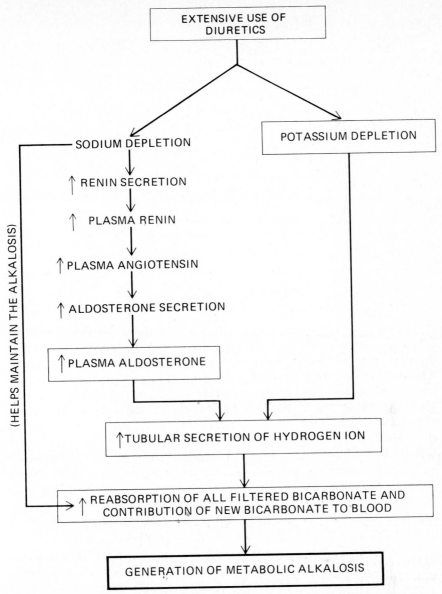

Figure 9-8 Pathway by which overuse of diuretics leads to a metabolic alkalosis. In contrast to the previous figure, the elevated aldosterone is not the cause of the potassium depletion. Note also that the salt depletion, via a nonaldosterone mechanism, helps to maintain the alkalosis once it has been generated.

exchanged for hydrogen ion across the luminal membrane. This fact makes it easy to visualize that, were hydrogen-ion secretion inhibited, sodium

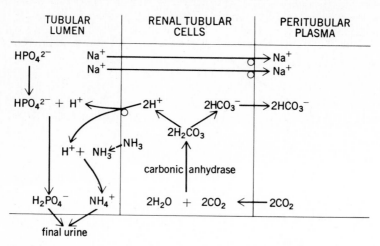

Figure 9-9 Tubular sodium-hydrogen ion "exchange" during formation of titratable acid and ammonium.

reabsorption would also decrease. Moreover, even in the distal nephron, which lacks direct sodium–hydrogen-ion coupling, sodium reabsorption is, in part, *indirectly* coupled by electrical forces to hydrogen-ion secretion. This indirect electrical coupling stems from the fact that bicarbonate ions constitute approximately 25 percent of the anions in the glomerular filtrate. Unless bicarbonate ions were reabsorbed at close to the same rate as sodium, there would occur a large separation of charge and a marked increase in the negativity of the tubular lumen — an event that would strongly retard further net sodium reabsorption. In fact, as we have seen, bicarbonate reabsorption normally occurs at the same rate as, or faster than, sodium reasbsorption; since the bicarbonate is reabsorbed as a result of hydrogen-ion secretion, there is, in a sense, the "exchange" of a secreted hydrogen ion for a reabsorbed sodium ion even in the absence of direct coupling.

This type of exchange occurs not only when the secreted hydrogen ion achieves bicarbonate reabsorption but also when the hydrogen ion is used in the formation of titratable acid and ammonium. In both cases the titration of HPO_4^{2-} to $H_2PO_4^-$ or of NH_3 to NH_4^+ produces a net gain of one positive charge in the lumen, thereby permitting a sodium ion to be reabsorbed simultaneously with no change in intraluminal charge (Fig. 9-9).

In effect, then, sodium is reabsorbed either with chloride or in exchange for hydrogen ion. There are several very important implications of these relationships for sodium chloride reabsorption:

1 There is usually an inverse correlation between the excretion rates of chloride and bicarbonate. Most simply viewed, when sodium reabsorption is proceeding relatively more rapidly than acid secretion and bicarbonate reabsorption, then more chloride will accompany the reabsorbed sodium (because of increased luminal negativity). Therefore, less chloride will be excreted. Conversely, when the rate of acid secretion is high enough so that filtrated bicarbonate is totally reabsorbed and large quantities of titratable acid and ammonium are formed, then less chloride is reabsorbed, since a larger fraction of the sodium is reabsorbed in exchange for hydrogen ion. Increased renal excretion of chloride is, therefore, one of the reasons that plasma chloride tends to go down during the renal compensation for a metabolic acidosis.

2 Whenever tubular acid secretion is inadequate to effect complete bicarbonate reabsorption, there is usually the obligatory excretion of some sodium in the urine along with the bicarbonate. However, the loss of sodium is usually not as great as the loss of bicarbonate, because (as we saw in the previous chapter) alkalosis induces increased potassium secretion, and the secretion of potassium ions into the lumen allows an equivalent amount of sodium to be reabsorbed with no change in intraluminal potential. An interesting example of this phenomenon is the renal response to administration of drugs that inhibit renal carbonic anhydrase. Inhibition of this enzyme reduces acid secretion, which in turn reduces bicarbonate reabsorption. The net result is an increased excretion of sodium, bicarbonate, and water. (Unreabsorbed solute always causes the excretion of increased amounts of water.) In addition, the inhibition of carbonic anhydrase alkalinizes the renal tubular cells. (The reason for this can be seen in Fig. 9-2a.) The increased intracellular pH induces an enhanced secretion of potassium so that a large fraction of the excreted bicarbonate is accompanied by potassium rather than by sodium.

Study questions: 64 to 72

CHAPTER 10

REGULATION OF CALCIUM BALANCE AND EXTRACELLULAR CONCENTRATION

OBJECTIVES

The student understands the regulation of calcium balance and extracellular concentration.

1 States the normal plasma calcium concentration and the percent that is protein-bound; states the effect of pH on the free and bound fractions
2 Describes the gastrointestinal handling of calcium; defines net calcium absorption and total calcium absorption
3 Describes the basic renal handling of calcium; states the effects of change in sodium intake and of metabolic acidosis on calcium excretion
4 States the percentage of total body calcium in bone
5 Lists the effects of parathyroid hormone and their adaptive value
6 Describes the control of secretion of parathyroid hormone
7 Describes the sequence of reactions leading from 7-dehydrocholesterol to $1,25\text{-}(OH)_2D_3$; states two major controls over the 1-hydroxylation step
8 Lists the effects of $1,25\text{-}(OH)_2D_3$
9 Defines calcitonin and states its suggested role in calcium regulation
10 Describes the direct and indirect effects of an increased plasma calcium concentration on renal calcium handling
11 Predicts changes in plasma and urinary calcium and phosphate in patients with hyperparathyroidism or with vitamin D deficiency

12 States the effects of cortisol and growth hormone on calcium balance

13 Describes the renal handling of phosphate; states two mechanisms that cause increased urinary phosphate excretion when dietary phosphate is elevated

Extracellular calcium concentration is normally maintained within very narrow limits, the requirement for precise regulation stemming primarily from the profound effects of calcium on neuromuscular excitability. A low calcium concentration increases the excitability of nerve and muscle cell membranes so that patients with diseases in which low calcium occurs suffer from *hypocalcemic tetany*, characterized by skeletal muscle spasms, which can be severe enough to cause death by asphyxia. Hypercalcemia is also dangerous because it causes cardiac arrhythmias as well as depressed neuromuscular excitability.

It is important to recognize that the plasma calcium (normally 5 meq/L or 2.5 mmol/L) exists in three general forms in approximately the following proportions: (1) 45 percent is in the ionized (Ca^{++}) form, the only biologically active form in nerve, muscle, and other target organs; (2) 15 percent is complexed to anions with relatively low molecular weights, such as citrate and phosphate; (3) 40 percent is reversibly bound to plasma proteins. One of the most important influences on binding is the plasma pH. An increase in pH causes increased calcium binding because the decreased acidity converts more of the protein to the anionic form; i.e., it exposes additional negatively charged binding sites. Thus, a patient with alkalosis is susceptible to tetany; whereas a patient with acidosis will not manifest tetany at levels of total plasma calcium low enough to cause symptoms in normal people.

EFFECTOR SITES FOR CALCIUM HOMEOSTASIS

Normally, the body remains in stable calcium balance; i.e., the amount of ingested calcium is equal to the calcium lost in the urine, feces, and sweat combined. However, in contrast to the situation for the other ions described in this book, the major variable homeostatically controlled to achieve this balance is the rate of gastrointestinal absorption. Our earlier chapters on ion and water homeostasis were concerned almost entirely with the renal handling of these substances. It was possible to do so for several reasons: (1) Although internal exchanges (between extracellular fluid, on the one hand, and bone and cells, on the other) are important for these substances, the major homeostatic controls act via the kidneys. (2) Absorption of these substances from the gut approximates 100 percent under normal circumstances and is not a major controlled variable. Neither of these statements holds true for calcium homeostasis. Accordingly, this section must deal not only with the renal handling of calcium but with the other two major effector sites for calcium homeostasis — bone and the gastronintestinal tract.

Gastrointestinal Tract

Net calcium absorption by the gastrointestinal tract is defined as the difference between dietary intake and fecal excretion. On a typical daily intake of 1000 mg, net calcium absorption is only approximately 100 mg, i.e., 10 percent of intake (contrast this to the virtually complete absorption of water and the other ions described in this book). The remaining 900 mg will appear in the feces. However, the situation is more complex than this, since the intestinal epithelium secretes a large quantity of endogenous calcium into the lumen.

$$
\begin{aligned}
\text{Ca ingested} &= 1000 \text{ mg/day} \\
\text{Ca secreted into intestinal lumen} &= \underline{600 \text{ mg/day}} \\
\text{Total in intestinal lumen} &= 1600 \text{ mg/day} \\
\text{Absorbed from gut} &= \underline{700 \text{ mg/day}} \\
\text{Excreted in feces} &= 900 \text{ mg/day}
\end{aligned}
$$

Thus in this example, 100 mg of new calcium is added to the blood each day; i.e., *net* calcium absorption is 10 percent of the ingested calcium, but *total* calcium absorption is actually 700 mg/day. Note that if gut absorption were reduced to 600 mg/day, then none of the ingested calcium would have been retained. Conversely, net calcium absorption could potentially be increased 10-fold (to 1000 mg/day) were total absorption raised to 1600 mg/day. Finally, lowering the rate of absorption to 500 mg/day would result in the fecal loss of 1100 mg/day; i.e., the person would go into negative calcium balance.

Such changes in absorption are, in fact, elicited when changes occur in dietary calcium or total body calcium balance. Indeed, the control of absorption constitutes, quantitatively, the major homeostatic process for maintaining calcium balance.

Kidney

The kidneys handle calcium by filtration and reabsorption. Only about 60 percent of the plasma calcium is filterable, the remainder being protein-bound. Reabsorption[1] occurs throughout the nephron, with the exception of the descending limb of Henle, and its quantitative pattern is similar to that of sodium: About 60 percent of the reabsorption occurs proximally,

---

[1] The cellular mechanisms of calcium reabsorption vary in different segments and are still not clearly worked out (see Suggested Readings).

and the remainder in the ascending limb of Henle, the distal tubule, and collecting tubules. Reabsorption normally approximates 98 to 99 percent, the 1 to 2 percent escaping reabsorption generally being equal to the normal net addition of new calcium to the body via the gastrointestinal tract (100 mg in our example). Thus, just as was true for the other ions discussed in this book, the kidneys help maintain a constant balance of total body calcium by matching output to intake; when intake is altered, the rate of excretion is homeostatically altered. However, the kidneys respond to changes in dietary calcium much less than they do to changes in sodium, water, or potassium. For example, it has been estimated that only about 5 percent of an increment in dietary calcium appears in the urine. This is because most of the dietary increment fails to be absorbed from the gastrointestinal tract. At the other end of the spectrum, when dietary intake of calcium is reduced to extremely low levels, there is a slow reduction of urinary calcium, but some continues to appear in the urine for weeks.

How do the renal homeostatic mechanisms operate? Since calcium is filtered and reabsorbed, but not secreted:

Ca excretion = Ca filtered − Ca reabsorbed

Accordingly, excretion can be altered homeostatically by changing either the filtered load or the rate of reabsorption. Both occur. For example, what happens when a person increases his calcium intake? Transiently, intake exceeds output, positive calcium balance ensues, and plasma calcium concentration increases. This in itself increases the filtered mass of calcium and increases excretion. Simultaneously, as we shall see, the increased plasma calcium triggers hormonal changes that cause a diminished reabsorption. The net result of these responses is increased calcium excretion.

A bewildering array of factors *not* designed to maintain calcium homeostasis can also influence urinary calcium excretion, mainly by stimulating or inhibiting tubular reabsorption. These include a large number of hormones, ions, acid-base disturbances, and drugs (see Suggested Readings). One of the most important of them is sodium. Under many circumstances, changes in calcium excretion can be induced simply by administering or withholding salt. (This fact is made use of clinically when one wishes to increase or decrease the amount of calcium in the body.) Indeed, changes in dietary sodium may be more effective in altering urinary calcium excretion than are changes in dietary calcium. Clearly, there is some kind of coupling between sodium reabsorption and calcium reabsorption, at least in the proximal tubule and loop of Henle. In contrast, these two ions can be dissociated in the more distal nephron segments, since their major hormonal controls—aldosterone (sodium) and parathyroid hormone (calcium)–stimulate distal reabsorption only of one ion without affecting the other.[2]

A second very important factor that influences tubular calcium reabsorption but is not designed to maintain calcium homeostasis is the presence of a chronic metabolic acidosis. The mechanism is not known, but an acidosis markedly inhibits calcium reabsorption and, hence, causes increased calcium excretion. (We shall see that the source of most of this calcium is bone.) A chronic metabolic alkalosis tends to do just the opposite—enhance calcium reabsorption and reduce excretion.

Bone

The activities of the gastrointestinal tract and the kidneys determine the net intake and output of calcium for the entire body and, thereby, the overall state of calcium balance. In contrast, interchanges of calcium between extracellular fluid and bone do not alter total body balance but, rather, the distribution of calcium within the body. Approximately 99 percent of the total body calcium is contained in bone, which is basically a collagen-protein framework upon which calcium phosphate (and other minerals) are deposited in a crystal structure known as *hydroxyapatite*. Bone is not a dead, fixed tissue; rather, it is cellular and well supplied with blood. Most important, it is continuously broken down (resorbed) and simultaneously re-formed under the influence of the bone cells. Thus, bone provides a huge potential source or sink for the withdrawal or deposit of calcium from extracellular fluid. We shall see that several hormones exert important effects on the deposition or resorption of bone calcium.

HORMONAL CONTROL OF EFFECTOR SITES

Parathyroid Hormone

All three of the effector sites described above are subject to direct or indirect control by a polypeptide hormone called parathyroid hormone, produced by the parathyroid glands. Parathyroid-hormone production is controlled directly by the calcium concentration of the extracellular fluid bathing the cells of these glands. Lower calcium concentration stimulates parathyroid-hormone production and release, and a higher concentration does just the opposite. It should be emphasized that extracellular calcium concentration acts directly upon the parathyroids without any intermediary hormones or nerves.

---

[2] An interesting indication of the differences in distal reabsorption of these two ions is the fact that thiazide diuretics inhibit distal sodium reabsorption but facilitate distal calcium reabsorption. In contrast, diuretics that act mainly in the proximal tubule and/or loop of Henle inhibit reabsorption of both ions.

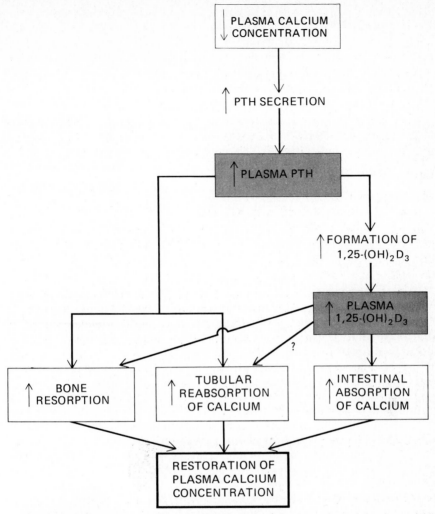

Figure 10-1 Hormonally mediated compensatory response to reduced plasma calcium concentration. PTH = parathyroid hormone. The effects of PTH and 1,25-(OH)$_2$D$_3$ on phosphate are not shown in the figure (see text and Fig. 10-2).

Parathyroid hormone exerts at least four distinct effects on calcium homeostasis (Figs. 10-1 and 10-2):

1 It increases the movement of calcium (and phosphate) from bone into extracellular fluid by stimulating bone resorption. In this manner the immense store of calcium contained in bone is made available for the regulation of extracellular calcium concentration.

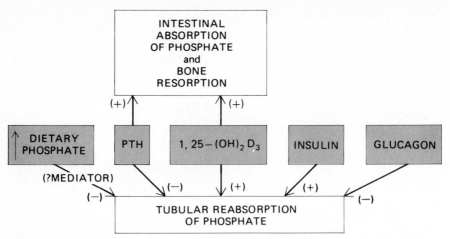

Figure 10-2 Effects of hormones and dietary phosphate on phosphate movements. (+) denotes a stimulation, and (−) and inhibition. Moreover, each (+) will tend to raise plasma phosphate concentration, whereas each (−) will tend to lower it.

2 It stimulates the activation of vitamin D (see below), and this latter hormone then increases intestinal absorption of calcium (and phosphate). Thus, the long-known ability of parathyroid hormone to stimulate intestinal absorption of these ions is not due to a direct action of it on the gut but rather is indirect and mediated by vitamin D.

3 It increases renal-tubular calcium reabsorption (by an action on the distal nephron) and thus decreases urinary calcium excretion. (Surprisingly, parathyroid hormone, at least in large doses, inhibits proximal-tubular reabsorption of calcium; even under such conditions, however, its stimulation of distal-tubular calcium reabsorption more than makes up for this proximal effect, and the overall nephron effect is, therefore, increased reabsorption.)

4 It reduces the renal tubular reabsorption of phosphate, thereby raising urinary phosphate excretion and lowering extracellular phosphate concentration. (Maximal amounts of parathyroid hormone can change the percent of filtered phosphate reabsorbed from 80 to 15 percent.)

The adaptive value of the first three effects should be obvious: They all result in a higher extracellular calcium concentration and thus compensate for the lower concentration, which originally stimulated parathyroid-hormone production. The adaptive value of the fourth effect can be understood in terms of both calcium and phosphate homeostasis. When parathyroid hormone induces bone resorption, both calcium and phosphate are released; similarly, its intestinal effect (via vitamin D) is to enhance the absorption of both calcium and phosphate. Accordingly, while the low calcium, which triggered the increase in parathyroid hormone, is being homeostatically compensated, the plasma phosphate would be raised above normal; the latter does not occur because of parathyroid hormone's inhibition of tubular phosphate reabsorption. Indeed, so potent is this effect that plasma phosphate may actually decrease when parathyroid-hormone levels are elevated. (This reduction in phosphate is adaptive in that it facilitates further bone resorption because of local interactions between calcium and phosphate.)

In contrast to the state described above, an increase in extracellular calcium concentration reduces parathyroid-hormone production and, thereby, produces increased urinary and fecal calcium loss and net movement of calcium from extracellular fluid into bone.

Parathyroid hormone has other functions in the body, but the four effects discussed above constitute the major mechanisms by which it integrates various organs and tissues in the regulation of extracellular calcium concentration. Another candidate to join these four was described in Chap. 9 — parathyroid hormone's inhibition of proximal-tubular hydrogen-ion secretion and, thereby, bicarbonate reabsorption. The result of this effect is an increased extracellular-fluid hydrogen-ion concentration (acidosis), which is known to displace calcium from plasma protein (as described above) and from bone; thus, free plasma calcium concentration rises. Whether this effect of parathyroid hormone is really important at physiological plasma levels of the hormone is still not settled.[3]

Hyperparathyroidism, due to a primary defect in the parathyroid glands (e.g., a hormone-secreting tumor),well illustrates the actions of parathyroid hormone. The excess hormone causes enhanced bone resorption, leading to bone thinning with the formation of completely calcium-free areas or cysts. Plasma calcium increases and plasma phosphate decreases; the latter is caused by increased urinary phosphate excretion. The increased plasma calcium is deposited in various body tissues, including the kidneys, where stones are formed. A seeming paradox is that urinary calcium excretion is increased. (Contrast this to the decreased calcium excretion induced by *physiological* amounts of parathyroid hormone — Fig. 10-1.) This occurs despite the fact that tubular calcium reabsorption is enhanced by parathyroid hormone. The explanation is that because of the elevated plasma calcium induced by parathyroid hormone, the filtered load of calcium increases even more than does reabsorptive rate — another excellent illustration of the necessity of taking both filtration and reabsorption into account when analyzing excretory changes.

Vitamin D

The term vitamin D denotes a group of closely related sterols. One of these compounds, called vitamin D_3 (or cholecalciferol), is formed by the action of ultraviolet radiation on 7-dehydrocholesterol in the skin. A second source of vitamin D is that ingested in food, and people, because of clothing and decreased out-of-doors living, are often dependent upon this dietary source. (The form of vitamin D found naturally in plants differs only trivially in

---

[3] It is likely that parathyroid hormone can induce a metabolic acidosis in ways other than its inhibition of tubular hydrogen-ion secretion. (See Suggested Readings.)

structure from vitamin D_3 and no distinction will be made between them in the subsequent description.)

Vitamin D_3 is inactive and must undergo metabolic changes within the body before it can influence its target cells. It enters the blood and is hydroxylated in the 25 position by the liver and then in the 1 position by the kidneys. The end result is the active form of vitamin $D-1,25$-dihydroxy vitamin D_3, abbreviated $1,25$-$(OH)_2D_3$. From this description, it should be evident that $1,25$-$(OH)_2D_3$ is actually a hormone, not a vitamin, since it is made in the body.

The major action of vitamin D is to stimulate active absorption of calcium (and phosphate) by the intestine. Thus, the major event in vitamin D deficiency is decreased gut calcium absorption, resulting in decreased plasma calcium. In children, the newly formed bone protein matrix fails to be calcified normally because of the low plasma calcium, leading to the disease *rickets*.

In addition to its effect on intestinal calcium absorption, vitamin D also significantly enhances bone resorption. The mechanism underlying this effect is unclear but may involve a facilitation by vitamin D of the bone-resorption effect exerted by parathyroid hormone. Finally, vitamin D can also stimulate the renal-tubular reabsorption of calcium (and phosphate), but whether this effect is significant physiologically remains unsettled.

The blood concentration of the active form of vitamin $D-1,25$-$(OH)_2D_3$ — is subject to physiological control. The major control point is the final hydroxylation step, which occurs in the kidneys. This step is stimulated by parathyroid hormone, a phenomenon which is highly adaptive, for it provides a mechanism for simultaneously altering the levels of these hormones in the same direction. Thus, a low plasma-calcium concentration stimulates the secretion of parathyroid hormone, which, in turn, enhances the activation of vitamin D, and both substances contribute to the restoration of the plasma calcium to normal (Fig. 9-3).[4]

Parathyroid hormone is not the only modulator of $1,25$-$(OH)_2D_3$ formation. Phosphate is another important one.[5] In this case, a decreased plasma phosphate stimulates formation. This is adaptive in terms of phosphate homeostasis—decreased phosphate stimulates formation of $1,25$-$(OH)_2D_3$, which then enhances phosphate absorption from the gut (and, possibly, its reabsorption by the renal tubules), with a resulting compensatory increase in plasma phosphate.

---

[4] In addition to its indirect effect, via stimulation of PTH secretion, on the formation of $1,25$-$(OH)_2D_3$, it is possible that a low calcium, per se, directly enhances this formation.

[5] Many other possible inputs are presently being studied. For example, it is likely that estrogen and prolactin also stimulate formation of $1,25$-$(OH)_2D_3$; this would be adaptive in assuring increasing gut absorption of calcium and phosphate during pregnancy.

Finally, the recognition that the kidneys perform the key hydroxylation step in the activation of vitamin D has clarified why patients with renal disease generally manifest a serious deficiency of vitamin D, even when they are given large amounts of precursors of $1,25\text{-}(OH)_2D_3$. The damaged kidneys are simply unable to perform the activation step normally, and the result is a marked decrease in intestinal absorption of calcium. In contrast, therapy with $1,25\text{-}(OH)_2D_3$ results in dramatic improvement.

Calcitonin

Yet a third hormone, calcitonin, has significant effects on plasma calcium. Calcitonin is a peptide hormone secreted by cells within the thyroid gland which surround, but are completely distinct from, the thyroxine-secreting follicles. The calcitonin-secreting cells are called, therefore, *parafollicular cells*. Calcitonin can lower plasma calcium, primarily by inhibiting bone resorption. Its secretion is controlled, in part, directly by the calcium concentration of the plasma supplying the thyroid gland; an increased calcium causes increased calcitonin secretion. Thus, this system has been suspected of constituting another feedback control over plasma calcium concentration. However, its overall contribution to calcium homeostasis is very minor compared to that of parathyroid hormone and vitamin D; indeed, thyroidectomized persons with no detectable plasma calcitonin have no significant alteration in their plasma calcium concentration. Accordingly, emphasis has shifted away from calcitonin as a regulator of plasma calcium and toward its possible roles in regulating other physiological activites (see Suggested Readings).

Other Hormones

Parathyroid hormone and vitamin D are the major hormones that participate in homeostatic responses to changes in calcium balance. However, several other hormones do influence calcium, so that changes in their rates of secretion can produce calcium imbalances. Thus, high levels of cortisol can induce negative calcium balance by depressing gut absorption of calcium while increasing its renal excretion. Growth hormone also increases urinary calcium excretion, but it simultaneously increases gut absorption. The net effect of these counterbalancing influences of growth hormone is usually a positive calcium balance.

OVERVIEW OF RENAL PHOSPHATE HANDLING

The renal handling of phosphate has been mentioned several times in this chapter and elsewhere in the book, but almost always in the context of other topics, such as sodium reabsorption or urine acidification. This short section serves to emphasize certain key aspects of renal phosphate handling, per se, since control of urinary phosphate excretion is a major pathway for the homeostatic regulation of total body phosphate balance.

Approximately 5 to 10 percent of plasma phosphate is protein-bound, so that 90 to 95 percent is filterable at the glomerulus. Normally, approximately 75 percent of this filtered phosphate is actively reabsorbed, mainly in the proximal tubule (in co-transport with sodium). There is probably also some small degree of phosphate reabsorption in sites beyond the proximal tubule. There is no conclusive evidence for significant tubular secretion of phosphate (although this remains controversial).

As with other substances handled by filtration and tubular reabsorption, the rate of phosphate excretion can be changed by altering the mass filtered per unit time and/or the mass reabsorbed per unit time. Because the reabsorptive T_m for phosphate is very close to the normal filtered load, even relatively small increases in plasma phosphate concentration (and, hence, filtered load) can produce relatively large increases in phosphate excretion. This is just what occurs when plasma phosphate concentration increases as a result of increased dietary phosphate intake.

But changes in filtered load are not the major reason that phosphate excretion increases or decreases homeostatically in response to altered dietary intake. Tubular reabsorption also changes. The observed facts are that a diet low in phosphate induces, over time, an increase in the rate of phosphate reabsorption (as well as an increase in the transport maximum for phosphate); a diet high in phosphate does just the opposite. These homeostatic adaptations are not due to changes in parathyroid hormone or vitamin D, and the pathways and mechanisms involved remain unknown.

To reiterate, changes in parathyroid hormone do not mediate the homeostatic association between dietary phosphate and tubular phosphate reabsorption. Nevertheless, as we have seen, whenever parathyroid hormone is increased or decreased, tubular phosphate reabsorption is powerfully inhibited or stimulated, respectively. Other hormones, too, are known to alter phosphate reabsorption; for example, insulin increases it and glucagon decreases it. These are only a few of the many factors that can influence phosphate reabsorption and, hence, phosphate excretion and balance.

Figure 10-2 summarizes some of the major controls over renal, bone, and gastrointestinal phosphate transport.

Study questions: 71 to 73

STUDY QUESTIONS

As emphasized in the preface, these questions do not cover the material of this book systematically or comprehensively; that is the function of the objectives at the beginning of each chapter. Rather, these questions provide practice and additional feedback in certain areas, particularly those which commonly give some difficulty.

Q-1 The difference between superficial and juxtamedullary nephrons is that the former have their glomeruli in the cortex whereas the glomeruli of the latter arise in the medulla. True or false?

A-1 False. All glomeruli are in the cortex. See text for description.

Q-2 When a patient is given a drug that inhibits angiotensin-converting enzyme, there is little physiological effect because the decrement in angiotensin II is compensated for by the simultaneous rise in angiotensin I. True or false?

A-2 False. Angiotensin II is much more potent than Angiotensin I.

Q-3 Substance T is present in the urine. Does this *prove* that it is filterable at the glomerulus?

A-3 No. It is a possibility, but there is another; substance T may be secreted by the tubules.

Q-4 Substance V is not normally present in the urine. Does this *prove* that it is neither filtered nor secreted?

A-4 No. It is a possibility, but there is another; V may be filtered and/or secreted, but all the V entering the lumen via these routes may be completely reabsorbed.

Q-5 The concentration of calcium in Bowman's capsule is 3 mM, whereas its plasma concentration is 5 mM. How do you explain this?

A-5 Approximately 40% of the calcium in plasma is bound to proteins and so is not filterable.

Q-6 The concentration of glucose in plasma is 100 mg/100 mL and the GFR is 125 mL/min. How much glucose is filtered per minute?

A-6 125 mg/min. The amount of *any* substance filtered per unit time is given by the product of the GFR and the filterable plasma concentration of the substance, in this case, 125 mL/min × 100 mg/100 mL.

Q-7 A protein has a molecular weight of 20,000 and a plasma concentration of 100 mg/L. The GFR is 100 L/day. How much of this protein is filtered per day?

A-7 No exact value can be calculated from the above data because the concentration of the protein in the glomerular filtrate is not known. The molecular weight is high enough so that some "sieving" would occur, but low enough so that the restriction would not be total.

Q-8 A drug is noted to cause a decrease in GFR. What might the drug be doing?

A-8 (a) Constricting glomerular mesangial cells and, hence, reducing K_f.
(b) Lowering arterial pressure and, hence, P_{GC}.
(c) Constricting the afferent arteriole and, hence, reducing P_{GC}.
(d) Dilating the efferent arteriole and, hence, reducing P_{GC}.
(e) Causing obstruction somewhere in the urinary system and, hence, increasing P_{BC}.
(f) Increasing plasma albumin concentration and, hence, π_{GC}.
(g) Decreasing the amount of blood flow to the kidneys, resulting in a steeper use of π_{GC} along the length of the glomerular capillaries.

Q-9 A drug is noted to cause an increase in GFR with no change in net filtration pressure. What must the drug be doing?

A-9 It must be increasing K_f, i.e., changing the hydraulic permeability of the glomerular membranes and/or the surface area available for filtration.

Q-10 Substance O is filtered, reabsorbed, and secreted. If you were designing a system for increasing the renal excretion of substance O when its intake is high, what could you do?

A-10 There are three possibilities (either alone or in combination): Increase filtered substance O by increasing either GFR or plasma concentration of substance O; inhibit tubular reabsorption of substance O; enhance tubular secretion of substance O.

Q-11 There is a net movement of anionic phosphate across the luminal membrane into the tubular cells even though cytosolic phosphate concentration is higher than luminal and there is a cytosol-negative potential difference across the luminal membrane. Does this prove that the phosphate movement is driven by the direct input of energy from splitting ATP?

A-11 No. It proves that the movement is active, but it could be a secondary active transport (and, in fact, is).

Q-12 You are trying to measure the reabsorptive T_m for glucose in a patient. You plan to calculate glucose reabsorption [(GFR $\times$ P_G)–($U_G \times V$)] as you raise plasma glucose stepwise by infusion. You stop the test when glucose first appears in the urine, assuming that the reabsorptive rate at this time equals the T_m. Is this correct?

A-12 No. Glucose starts to appear in the urine *before* the T_m for all nephrons has been reached. Therefore, if you had continued to raise plasma glucose, reabsorptive rate would have increased some more. You can be certain that T_m has been reached only when the reabsorptive rate remains constant despite another increment in plasma glucose.

Q-13 The hospital lab reports that your patient's creatinine clearance is 120g/day. This value is:
a Normal
b Significantly below normal
c Nonsense

A-13 c. Clearance units are volume per time, not mass per time.

Q-14 The following test results were obtained on specimens from a person over a 2-h period during infusion of inulin and PAH.

$$\text{Total urine vol} = 0.14L$$
$$U_{In} = 100 \text{ mg}/100 \text{ mL}$$
$$P_{In} = 1 \text{ mg}/100 \text{ mL}$$
$$U_{urea} = 220 \text{ mmol/L}$$
$$P_{urea} = 5 \text{ mmol/L}$$
$$U_{PAH} = 700\text{mg/mL}$$
$$P_{PAH} = 2\text{mg/mL}$$
$$\text{Hematocrit} = 0.40$$

What are the clearances of inulin, urea, and PAH? What is the effective renal plasma flow (ERPF)? What is the effective renal blood flow (ERBF)? How much urea is reabsorbed? How much PAH is secreted (assuming no PAH reabsorption and complete filterability of PAH)?

A-14

$$C_{\text{In}} = \frac{U_{\text{In}}V}{P_{\text{In}}}$$

$$= \frac{100 \text{ mg}/100 \text{ mL} \times 0.14 \text{ L}/2 \text{ h}}{1 \text{ mg}/100 \text{ mL}}$$

$$= 14.0 \text{ L}/2 \text{ h}; \text{ this is the GFR}$$

$$C_{\text{urea}} = \frac{U_{\text{urea}}V}{P_{\text{urea}}}$$

$$= \frac{220 \text{ mmol}/L \times 0.14 \text{ L}/2 \text{ h}}{5 \text{ mmol}/L}$$

$$= 6.16 \text{ L}/2 \text{ h}$$

$$C_{\text{PAH}} = \frac{U_{\text{PAH}}V}{P_{\text{PAH}}}$$

$$= \frac{700 \text{ mg}/\text{mL} \times 0.14 \text{ L}/2 \text{ h}}{2 \text{ mg}/\text{mL}}$$

$$= 49.0 \text{ L}/2 \text{ h}$$

$$\text{ERPF} = 49.0 \text{ L}/2 \text{ h}$$

$$\text{ERBF} = 81.7 \text{ L}/2 \text{ h}$$

$$\text{Reabsorbed urea} = \text{filtered urea} - \text{excreted urea}$$

$$= (14.0 \text{ L}/2 \text{ h} \times 5 \text{ mmol}/L)$$

$$-(220 \text{ mmol}/L \times 0.14 \text{ L}/2 \text{ h})$$

$$= 39.2 \text{ mmol}/2 \text{ h}$$

$$\text{PAH secreted} = \text{PAH excreted} - \text{PAH filtered}$$

$$= (700 \text{ mg}/\text{mL} \times 0.14 \text{ L}/2 \text{ h})$$

$$-(2 \text{ mg}/\text{mL} \times 14.0 \text{ L}/2 \text{ h})$$

$$= 98.0 \text{ g}/2 \text{ h} - 28.0 \text{ g}/2 \text{ h}$$

$$= 70.0 \text{ g}/2 \text{ h}$$

Q-15 In the above problem, you also obtained a sample of plasma from a renal vein. Its PAH concentration was 0.2 mg/mL. What is the true renal plasma flow?

A-15 54.4 L

$$\text{TRPF} = \frac{U_{\text{PAH}}V}{P_{\text{PAH}} - \text{renal venous}_{\text{PAH}}}$$

$$= \frac{700 \text{ mg}/\text{mL} \times 0.14 \text{ L}/2 \text{ h}}{2 \text{ mg}/\text{mL} - 0.2 \text{ mg}/\text{mL}}$$

$$= 54.4 \text{ L}/2 \text{ h}$$

Q-16 Now that you know that the renal venous plasma contained PAH, was the value you calculated for secreted PAH the secretory T_m for PAH?

A-16 No. There is always PAH in the renal venous plasma, mainly because some of the renal blood flow does not pass near proximal tubules. The way to do a PAH secretory T_m is to keep raising the systemic plasma PAH by infusion and when the mass of PAH secreted (calculated just as you did in the problem) stops increasing with further increments in systemic plasma PAH, that mass is the T_m.

Q-17 An increase in the plasma concentration of inulin causes which of the following in the renal clearance of inulin:
a Increase
b Decrease
c No change

A-17 c. $C_{In} = U_{In}V/P_{In}$. When P_{In} increases, there is no change in C_{In} because U_{In} rises an identical amount. In other words, the mass of inulin filtered and excreted increases but the volume of plasma supplying this inulin, i.e., completely cleared of inulin, is unaltered.

Q-18 The clearance of substance A is less than that simultaneously determined for inulin. Give three possible explanations.

A-18 (1) Substance A is, itself, a large molecule poorly filtered at the glomerulus.
(2) Substance A is bound, at least in part, to plasma protein.
(3) Substance A is reabsorbed.

Q-19 List in order of decreasing renal clearance the following substances:
Glucose
Urea
Sodium
Inulin
Creatinine
PAH

A-19 PAH
Creatinine
Inulin
Urea
Sodium
Glucose

Q-20 The following test results were obtained during a clearance experiment.

$$U_{In} = 50 \text{ mg/L}$$
$$P_{In} = 1 \text{ mg/L}$$
$$V = 2 \text{ mL/min}$$
$$U_{Na} = 75 \text{ m}M$$
$$P_{Na} = 150\text{m}M$$

What is the fractional excretion (FE) of sodium?

A-20 0.01

$$FE_{Na} = \frac{\text{mass Na excreted}}{\text{mass Na filtered}} = \frac{U_{Na}V}{GFR \times P_{Na}} = \frac{U_{Na}V}{C_{In} \times P_{Na}}$$
$$= \frac{75 \text{ mmol/L} \times 2 \text{ ml/min}}{100 \text{ ml/min} \times 150 \text{ mmol/L}}$$
$$= 0.01$$

This means that only 1% of the filtered sodium was excreted; i.e., 99% was reabsorbed.

A second completely equivalent way of calculating FE would be to use the " double" ratio:

$$FE_{Na} = \frac{U_{Na}/P_{Na}}{U_{In}/P_{In}} = \frac{75 \text{ m}M/150 \text{ m}M}{50 \text{ mg/L}/1 \text{ mg/L}}$$

Q-21 During a micropuncture experiment, a sample of tubular fluid (TF) was obtained from the end of the proximal tubule and its inulin concentration was found to be twice as high as the concentration in plasma, i.e. ($TF_{In}/P_{In} = 2$). How much water was reabsorbed by the proximal tubule?

A-21 50% of the water that was originally filtered. Since inulin is neither reabsorbed nor secreted, its rise in concentration along the nephron is due entirely to water reabsorption and can, therefore, be used to calculate the extent of water reabsorption.

Q-22 If 50 percent of a person's nephrons were destroyed, which of the following compounds would be likely to show an increased blood concentration?

a Urea
b Creatinine

c Uric acid
d Most amino acids
e Glucose
f Purines

A-22 a,b,c. These waste products are all normally excreted in large amounts; a decreased GFR would cause their plasma concentrations to increase until filtered load was increased enough to reestablish normal excretion. In contrast, the reabsorption T_ms for glucose, amino acids, purines, and many other organic compounds that are not waste products are usually so high as to prevent significant excretion. Accordingly, their plasma concentrations are virtually independent of renal function; i.e., the kidneys do not participate in the setting of their plasma concentrations.

Q-23 A month after 80 percent of the nephrons are destroyed, what will the blood-urea concentration be, assuming it was 5 mmol/L before the disease occurred?
a 25 mmol/L
b 5 mmol/L
c 6 mmol/L
d Continuously rising
e Not calculable unless it is assumed that the patient's protein intake did not change as a result of the disease

A-23 e. If one assumes a constant protein intake, then 25 mmol/L would have been the correct answer, since total filtered urea could be restored to normal at this point [25(0.2 × 180) = 5 × 180]. However, had protein intake been reduced by 50 percent, then plasma urea would stabilize at 12.5 mmol/L, since only 50 percent as much urea would be produced.

Q-24 The concentration of urea in urine is always much higher than the concentration in plasma. Is this because the overall tubular handling of urea is secretion?

A-24 No. The overall tubular handling of urea is reabsorption; i.e., reabsorption is far more extensive in the proximal tubule and collecting ducts than secretion is in the loops of Henle. The reason urinary urea concentration is higher than that of plasma is that relatively more water has been reabsorbed than urea, thereby concentrating the urea in the tubule.

Q-25 If the concentration of protein in the glomerular filtrate was 0.005 g/100 mL and none was reabsorbed, how much protein would be excreted per day (assuming a normal GFR)?

A-25   9g

$$\text{Excreted} = \text{filtered} - \text{reabsorbed}$$
$$= (0.05 \text{ g/L} \times 180 \text{ L/day}) - 0$$
$$= 9 \text{ g/day}$$

Q-26   A drug has been found to increase uric acid excretion. Give at least three ways it might act.

A-26   (1) Increase uric acid synthesis → increased plasma uric acid → increased filtration
(2) Stimulation of secretion
(3) Inhibition of reabsorption

Q-27   If you wished to increase your patient's excretion of quinine, a weak organic base, what change in urinary pH would you try to induce?

A-27   Decreased pH. This would convert more of the quinine to its charged form and prevent its passive reabsorption.

Q-28   During a dog experiment, a clamp around the renal artery is partially tightened so as to reduce renal arterial pressure from a mean of 120 mmHg to 80 mmHg. How much do you predict RBF will change?
a 33% decrease
b Zero
c 5 to 10% decrease
d 33% increase

A-28   c. Autoregulation prevents the RBF from decreasing in direct proportion to mean arterial pressure, but autoregulation is not 100%.

Q-29   A patient suffers a hemorrhage which drops the mean arterial pressure by 25%. What do you predict happens to the GFR and RBF?
a Almost no change
b A fairly large decrease, RBF > GFR

A-29   b. If you answered "a," you probably assumed that autoregulation would prevent any significant change. This is wrong because the drop in pressure reflexly stimulates increased sympathetic tone to the kidney (and increased plasma angiotensin II). (See text for the reason the GFR change is less than the RBF change.)

Q-30   A normal dog is given a drug that inhibits sodium chloride reabsorption by the ascending loop of Henle. GFR decreases within seconds to a particular value and then slowly decreases even more over the next 2 h. Why?

A-30 The immediate decrease in GFR is due to tubulo-glomerular feedback; the more delayed additional decrease is due to reflexly increased sympathetic outflow to the kidney, triggered by the progressive diuretic-induced depletion of body sodium and water.

Q-31 In the situation described in question 29, what would happen to RBF
(relative to its value following the hemorrhage) if the hemorrhaged
person were given a drug that blocks synthesis of prostaglandins?
a increase
b remain the same
c decrease

A-31 c. Increased sympathetic outflow and increased angiotensin II induce
the synthesis of vasodilator prostaglandins; the drug would prevent
this and, hence, eliminate the usual prostaglandin-dependent oppo-
sition to renal vasoconstriction.

Q-32 A dog is subjected to a mild hemorrhage; its mean arterial pressure decreases slightly, and its plasma renin concentration increases
markedly. It is then given a drug that blocks beta-adrenergic receptors. Its plasma renin decreases back toward the normal (pre-
hemorrhage) values but still remains elevated to some extent. Why?

A-32 Most of the stimulus for increased renin release in this situation
was via the renal sympathetic nerves and epinephrine, which act
on the granular cells via beta-adrenergic receptors. Some stimulus
still remains, however, via the intrarenal baroreceptors and macula
densa.

Q-33 A normal person is given a drug that blocks angiotensin-converting
enzyme. What happens to renin secretion?

A-33 It increases. Angiotensin II exerts a potent inhibitory effect on
renin secretion; therefore, eliminating angiotensin II relieves this
inhibition, resulting in more renin secretion.

Q-34 In the steady state, what is the amount of sodium chloride excreted
daily in the urine by a normal person ingesting 12 g of sodium
chloride per day?
a 12 g/day
b Less than 12 g/day

A-34 b. Urinary excretion in the steady state must be less than ingested
sodium chloride by an amount equal to that lost in the sweat and
feces. This is normally quite small, less than 1 g/day, so that urine
excretion in this case equals approximately 11 g/day.

Q-35 A person's plasma sodium concentration is 144 mmol/L; inulin clearance, 120 mL/min; urine volume, 36 mL in 30 min; and the urine sodium concentration, 200 mmol/L. What percent of filtered sodium is excreted?

A-35 1.4%

$$\text{Filtered Na}^+ = 144 \text{ mmol/L} \times 0.12 \text{ L/min}$$
$$= 17.28 \text{ mmol/min}$$
$$\text{Excreted Na}^+ = 0.036 \text{ L/30 min} \times 200 \text{ mmol/L}$$
$$= 0.24 \text{ mmol/min}$$
$$\% \frac{\text{Excreted}}{\text{Filtered}} = \frac{0.24}{17.28} \times 100 = 1.4\%$$

Q-36 In chronic renal disease, plasma urea may become markedly elevated. Under such circumstances urea will act as an osmotic diuretic. What does this do to sodium, chloride, and water excretion?

A-36 Sodium, chloride, and water excretion will all increase.

Q-37 Normally there are no *passive* fluxes of sodium into or out of the proximal tubule. True or false?

A-37 False. There are very large passive fluxes in both directions. However, there is little *net* passive flux because of the absence of a significant electrochemical gradient for sodium.

Q-38 **a** Complete inhibition of active chloride transport by the ascending loop of Henle would virtually eliminate the ability to excrete a concentrated urine. True or false?
b Increasing the passive permeability of the ascending loop to chloride would reduce the maximal concentrating ability of the kidney. True or false?
c Active reabsorption of sodium by the descending loop is a component of the countercurrent multiplier system. True or false?

A-38 (*a*) True.
(*b*) True. The gradient between ascending loop and interstitium at any *horizontal* level would be decreased; therefore the gradient from top to bottom would be decreased.
(*c*) False. There is no reabsorption of sodium (or chloride) by the descending loop.

Q-39 A normal experimental animal is given a drug, and a sample of tubular fluid (TF) is later collected by micropuncture from the end of the proximal convoluted tubule along with a plasma (P) sample. The TF/P ratio for inulin is 1.5 and for sodium is 0.99. Has the drug inhibited, stimulated, or done nothing to proximal sodium reabsorption?

A-39 Inhibited it. The inulin data reveal that only 30 percent of filtered water has been reabsorbed. Since TF/P for sodium is essentially unity (the normal value for proximal fluid), this means that only 30 percent of the filtered sodium was reabsorbed, a value far below normal.

Q-40 True or false questions.
   a Net reabsorption of sodium occurs in the ascending loop of Henle.
   b Net reabsorption of water occurs in the descending loop.
   c Net reabsorption of water occurs in the collecting ducts.
   d Net bulk flow of interstitial fluid into the vasa recta occurs.

A-40 All are true. The last may have given you trouble. The fact is that the vasa recta act as countercurrent exchangers to eliminate net overall *diffusion* of sodium and water into or out of the vasa recta by balancing any net movements in the descending vessels with opposite ones in the ascending. Thus, net diffusional movements are minimal, but normal capillary *bulk flow* must still be occurring, or otherwise the sodium and water reabsorbed from the loops of Henle and collecting ducts would not be carried away.

Q-41 A drug is given which blocks sodium channels or carriers in the luminal membrane all along the nephron but does not act on the Na-K-dependent ATPase in the basolateral membrane. What happens to sodium reabsorption?

A-41 It markedly decreases or ceases completely. Even though the active step is not altered by the drug, there will be little or no sodium entering the cell to be acted upon by the pumps.

Q-42 A drug is given which blocks all Na-K-dependent ATPase sites in the nephron. Would this eliminate chloride reabsorption in all nephron segments except the ascending loop of Henle?

A-42 Chloride reabsorption would be blocked everywhere, including the ascending loop of Henle. The active process for chloride in this latter segment is by co-transport with sodium.

Q-43 A patient taking large quantities of aspirin for arthritis manifests an unusually persistent degree of water retention. Why might this be?

A-43   Aspirin inhibits prostaglandin synthesis; therefore, the person is hyperresponsive to ADH, since ADH's partial inhibition of its own action, via stimulation of prostaglandin synthesis, is lost.

Q-44   In an experiment a dog's rate of glomerular filtration of sodium is found to be 15 mmol/min.
a How much sodium do you predict remains in the tubule at the end of the proximal tubule?
b Its GFR is suddenly increased by 33%. How much sodium now is left at the end of the proximal tubule?

A-44   (*a*) 5 mmol/min. Approximately two-thirds of filtered sodium is reabsorbed by the proximal tubule.
(*b*) 6.6 mmol/min. Filtered sodium rises from 15 to 20 mmol/min. Glomerulotubular balance maintains fractional sodium reabsorption at approximately two-thirds of the filtered load.

Q-45   Normally aldosterone controls the reabsorption of approximately 33 g of sodium chloride per day. If a patient loses 100 percent of adrenal function, will 33 g of sodium chloride be excreted per day indefinitely?

A-45   No. As soon as the patient starts to become sodium-deficient as a result of the increased sodium excretion, the usual sodium-retaining reflexes will be set into motion. They will, of course, be unable to raise aldosterone secretion, but they will lower GFR and alter the other factors that influence tubular sodium reabsorption so as to at least partially compensate for the decreased aldosterone-dependent sodium reabsorption.

Q-46   What happens to sodium excretion during quiet standing?
A-46   It decreases. Because of venous pooling of blood and increased filtration of fluid across the leg capillaries, quiet standing causes an effective decrease in plasma volume, which triggers all the described inputs leading to decreased sodium excretion (decreased GFR and increased tubular reabsorption).

Q-47   A patient has just suffered a severe hemorrhage and the plasma protein concentration is normal. (Not enough time has elapsed for interstitial fluid to move into the plasma.) Does this mean that the peritubular-capillary oncotic pressure is also normal?

A-47   No. It will probably be above normal because of an increased filtration fraction secondary to sympathetically mediated renal arteriolar constriction.

Q-48 If the right renal artery becomes abnormally constricted, what will happen to renin secretion by it and by the left kidney?

A-48 The right kidney has an increased secretion because of the decreased renal perfusion acting via the intrarenal baroreceptor and macula densa. This increased secretion will result in elevated systemic angiotensin II and arterial blood pressure, both of which will inhibit renin secretion from the left kidney.

Q-49 A patient with leaky glomeruli but normal tubules loses protein in the urine and, therefore, has a plasma albumin of 2.5 g/100 mL. Virtually all sodium ingested is retained (i.e., urinary excretion of sodium is close to zero) and the patient is becoming edematous. What is the stimulus for renal sodium retention in this case, since total extracellular volume is clearly greater than normal?

A-49 Because of the low plasma albumin, *plasma volume is decreased* as a result of the abnormal balance of forces across capillaries. This decreased plasma volume initiated sodium-retaining reflexes just as if the plasma volume had been decreased by diarrhea, a burn, etc. The retained fluid does not restore the plasma volume to normal, however, but merely filters into the interstitium, where it increases the edema. Interestingly, tubular sodium reabsorption is increased in this state despite the fact that peritubular-capillary protein concentration is almost certainly lower than normal, which should reduce tubular sodium reabsorption. A reflexly increased aldosterone level is certainly important in stimulating sodium reabsorption and overriding this effect of the low protein. Changes in renal hemodynamics and in the postulated natriuretic hormone may also be important.

Q-50 A patient is suffering from primary hyperaldosteronism, i.e., increased secretion of aldosterone, usually caused by an aldosterone-producing adrenal tumor. Is plasma renin concentration higher or lower than normal?

A-50 Lower. The increased aldosterone causes positive sodium balance, which reflexly inhibits renin secretion. Thus, one observes a high plasma aldosterone and a low plasma renin — a strong tip-off as to the presence of the disease, since in almost all other situations renin and aldosterone change in the same direction (because renin-angiotensin is the major control of aldosterone secretion).

Q-51 Any agent that increases sodium and water excretion is called a diuretic (even though natriuretic is probably a better term). List possible mechanisms of actions of these drugs.

A-51   (1) Increase GFR either by raising blood pressure or by dilating renal afferent arterioles.

(2) The above hemodynamic changes would also inhibit sodium reabsorption by increasing peritubular-capillary hydraulic pressure and/or reducing peritubular-capillary oncotic pressure (because of decreased filtration fraction).

(3) Directly inhibit the active-transport system for sodium, e.g., by blocking Na-K-dependent ATPase.

(4) Directly block chloride reabsorption in the thick ascending limb of Henle.

(5) Inhibit secretion of renin or aldosterone.

(6) Block action of aldosterone.

(7) Act as an osmotic diuretic by its osmotic contribution (mannitol, for example).

(8) Inhibit sodium–hydrogen-ion countertransport.

(9) Inhibit other hydrogen-ion secretory pathways. (You will not know this now, but will by the end of the book.)

This list is by no means exhaustive but does include the major clinically useful types of diuretics.

Q-52   A normal subject loses 2 L of isotonic salt solution because of diarrhea. He or she simultaneously drinks 2 L or pure water. What happens to:

a Extracellular-fluid volume

b Body-fluid osmolarity

c Renin and aldosterone secretion

d ADH secretion

A-52   (*a*) and (*b*) Extracellular volume and osmolarity both decrease. The entire 2 L of solution was lost from the extracellular compartment, since it was isotonic. (Therefore, osmolarity did not change, and no water moved into or out of cells.) The 2 L of ingested pure water is distributed throughout the body water, only about one-third remaining in the extracellular fluid. Moreover, the addition of pure water lowers the osmolarity.

(*c*) Increases, because of reflexes induced by the decreased extracellular volume.

(*d*) Cannot predict for certain but probably decreases. The decreased extracellular volume reflexly stimulates ADH secretion, but the reduced osmolarity should inhibit it via the hypothalamic osmoreceptors. The osmoreceptor input usually predominates during such "conflicts" unless the extracellular-volume depletion is very large.

Q-53 A person excretes 2 L of urine having an osmolarity of 600 mosmol/L. As a result, does body-fluid osmolarity *increase* or *decrease*? The change would be identical to that produced by *adding or substracting how many* liters of pure water?

A-53 Decrease; adding 2 L. He or she has excreted 2 L × 600 mosmol/L = 1200 mosmol total solute and 2 L water. Two liters of normal body fluids contain 2 L × 300 mosmol/L = 600 mosmol solutes. Accordingly, he or she has excreted 1200 − 600 = 600 mosmol pure solute beyond that needed for isotonicity. This will reduce the body-fluid osmolarity by an amount equivalent to that produced by adding 2 L pure water; i.e., 2 L of "free water" are retained.

Q-54 A person excreted 3 L of urine having an osmolarity of 150 mosmol/L. As a result, does body-fluid osmolarity *increase* or *decrease*? The change is identical to that produced by *adding or subtracting how many* liters pure water to/or from the body?

A-54 Increase; subtracting 1.5 L. He or she has excreted 3 L × 150 mosmol/L = 450 mosmol total solute, and 3 L water have been excreted. This amount of solute is contained in 450 mosmol ÷ 300 mosmol/L = 1.5 L normal body fluid. Therefore he or she has excreted 3 L − 1.5 L = 1.5 L "free water" from the body, thereby raising its osmolarity.

Q-55 What are the major renal sites of action of the following hormones?
Aldosterone
ADH
Renin
Epinephrine
Angiotensin II

A-55 Aldosterone: Late distal tubule and collecting duct
ADH: Late distal tubule and collecting duct
Renin: No renal site of action
Epinephrine: Renal arterioles, JG apparatus, and renal tubules
Angiotensin II: Renal arterioles and renal tubules

Q-56 What are the major controls of aldosterone secretion rate?
A-56 (1) Angiotensin II
(2) ACTH
(3) Plasma sodium concentration
(4) Plasma potassium concentration

Q-57 What are the major controls of renin secretion?

A-57   (1) Afferent-arteriolar pressure (intrarenal-baroreceptor)
(2) Sodium chloride load to the macula densa
(3) Activity of renal sympathetic nerves
(4) Angiotensin II

Q-58   What are the major controls of ADH secretion?
A-58   (1) Body-fluid osmolarity via hypothalamic osmoreceptors (or Na receptors)
(2) Plasma volume (specifically left atrial pressure via baroreceptors)

Q-59   Control of potassium excretion is achieved mainly by regulating the rate of:
a Potassium filtration
b Potassium reabsorption
c Potassium secretion
A-59   c

Q-60   A person in previously normal potassium balance maintains neurotic hyperventilation for several days. During this period what happens to potassium balance?
A-60   It becomes negative. The hyperventilation causes alkalosis, which in turn induces increased secretion of potassium (probably due to an alkalosis-induced elevation of renal-tubular-cell potassium concentration).

Q-61   A patient has a tumor in the adrenal which continuously secretes large quantities of aldosterone (primary hyperaldosteronism). Is the rate of potassium excretion normal, high, or low?
A-61   High. The increased aldosterone stimulates potassium secretion and, thereby, excretion. Moreover, once enough sodium has been retained to cause partial inhibition of proximal and loop sodium reabsorption, the increased delivery of fluid to the distal nephron further enhances potassium secretion. There is no potassium escape similar to the sodium escape from aldosterone.

Q-62   A patient with severe congestive heart failure is secreting large quantities of aldosterone. Is the rate of potassium excretion normal, high, or low?
A-62   Relatively normal. You may well have answered "high" assuming that the increased aldosterone would stimulate potassium secretion, as in the previous question. However, this effect is more than balanced by the fact that the patient has a diminished flow of fluid

into the distal tubule (because of increased proximal and loop reabsorption); recall that potassium secretion is greatly impaired when
the amount of fluid flowing through the distal tubule is reduced.
This explains why patients with the diseases of secondary hyperaldosteronism with edema do not lose large quantities of potassium,
whereas patients with primary hyperaldosteronism do.

Q-63 Give three reasons why osmotic diuresis (as, for example, in uncontrolled diabetic ketoacidosis) enhances potassium excretion.

A-63 (1) It inhibits potassium reabsorption.
(2) It increases fluid delivery to the distal tubule, resulting in
increased potassium secretion.
(3) It causes sodium depletion, which increases aldosterone secretion
(via the renin-angiotensin system), and this hormone stimulates
potassium secretion.

Q-64 A patient is observed to excrete 2 L of alkaline (pH = 7.6) urine
having a bicarbonate concentration of 28 mmol/L. The rate of
titratable-acid excretion is:
a 56 mmol
b Negative
c Cannot tell without data for ammonium

A-64 b. If the urine has a pH greater than 7.4, then clearly there is no
titratable acid (t.a.) excreted; indeed, there is negative t.a. excretion.
Ammonium does not contribute to t.a. and may be ignored in the
calculation of t.a.

Q-65 The following data are obtained for a subject:

$$C_{In} = 170 \text{ L/day}$$
$$P_{HCO_3^-} = 25 \text{ mmol/L}$$
$$U_{HCO_3^-} = 0$$
$$\text{Urine pH} = 5.8$$
$$\text{Titratable acid} = 26 \text{ mmol/day}$$
$$\text{Urine } NH_4^+ = 48 \text{ mmol/day}$$

Calculate:
a Total hydrogen ion secreted
b New bicarbonate added to the blood, i.e., acid excreted

A-65 (a) 4324 mmol/day. (Sum of HCO_3^- reabsorbed, t.a. excreted, and
NH_4^+ excreted.)
(b) 74 mmol/day. (Sum of t.a. and NH_4^+.)

Q-66   Which values could you predict are those for a patient with primary hyperaldosteronism?

	Urine pH	Plasma pH
a	6.9	7.55
b	8.2	7.55
c	4.8	7.30

A-66   a. This patient secretes excessive amounts of aldosterone, which induces potassium deficiency (because of increased renal potassium secretion). The potassium deficiency and aldosterone together then induce inappropriately large renal hydrogen-ion secretion, thereby producing a metabolic alkalosis. Note that the urine is still acid; i.e., the kidneys are not compensating.

Q-67   What are the three direct effects of aldosterone on the late distal tubule and collecting ducts?

A-67   Increased sodium reabsorption, increased potassium secretion, and increased hydrogen-ion secretion.

Q-68   A patient has been losing large amounts of HCl because of persistent vomiting for 3 days and, therefore, has a plasma pH of 7.50. The urine pH was 8.0 at the end of day one and 6.9 at the end of day three. Explain.

A-68   The alkaline urine on day one is the appropriate renal compensation for vomiting-induced alkalosis. The slightly acid urine on day three signifies that the kidneys are no longer compensating for alkalosis. This happens mainly because the progressive development of severe salt depletion stimulates proximal hydrogen-ion secretion, preventing loss of bicarbonate in the urine. (Potassium depletion and increased aldosterone may also contribute.)

Q-69   If renal-tubular carbonic anhydrase were completely inhibited, you would expect increased excretion of which of the following?
a Sodium
b Water
c Chloride
d Bicarbonate
e Ammonium
f Potassium

A-69   a, b, d, and f. See text for explanation of these increases. If anything, chloride excretion will decrease because of the reciprocal relationship between bicarbonate and chloride reabsorption. Ammonium excretion will be close to nil because the alkalinity of the tubular fluid minimizes diffusion trapping of ammonia.

Q-70 Match the top column with the bottom column. ("Increased" or "decreased" is with reference to normal.)
 a Diabetic ketoacidosis
 b Hypoventilation
 c Excessive ingestion of sodium bicarbonate
 1. Increased plasma pH, increased plasma bicarbonate, alkaline urine
 2. Decreased plasma pH, decreased plasma bicarbonate, acidic urine
 3. Decreased plasma pH, increased plasma bicarbonate, acidic urine

A-70 (a) 2
 (b) 3
 (c) 1

Q-71 Which of the following would you expect to find in a patient suffering from primary hypersecretion of parathyroid hormone?
 a Increased plasma calcium
 b Decreased plasma phosphate
 c Increased urine calcium
 d Increased tubular reabsorption of calcium
 e Increased urine phosphate
 f Increased plasma calcitonin
 g Increased plasma $1,25-(OH)_2D_3$

A-71 All are correct. c and d are not mutually exclusive because of the marked increase in filtered calcium. Calcitonin is reflexly increased by the increased plasma calcium. Formation of $1,25-(OH)_2D_3$ is enhanced by parathyroid hormone and by the decreased plasma phosphate as well.

Q-72 Which of the following would you expect to find in a person whose kidneys could not synthesize $1,25-(OH)_2D_3$?
 a Decreased gastrointestinal absorption of calcium
 b Decreased gastrointestinal absorption of phosphate
 c Decreased plasma-calcium concentration
 d Increased plasma-parathyroid-hormone concentration

A-72 All. The increased parathyroid hormone secretion is stimulated by the low plasma calcium.

Q-73 Complete inhibition of active sodium reabsorption would cause an increase in the excretion of which of the following substances?

     a Water
     b Urea
     c Chloride
     d Glucose
     e Amino acids
     f Potassium
     g Bicarbonate
     h Calcium

A-73 All. The reasons are all given in relevant sections of the text.

SUGGESTED READINGS

RESEARCH TECHNIQUES

Burg, M.: Introduction: Background and Development of Microperfusion Technique, *Kidney Int.,* **22**:417 (1982).

Burg, M., and J. Orloff: Perfusion of Isolated Renal Tubules, in R. W. Berliner and J. Orloff (eds.), "Handbook of Renal Physiology," sec. 8, American Physiological Society, Wash., D.C., 1973.

Gottschalk, C. W., and W. E. Lassiter: Micropuncture Methodology, in R. W. Berliner and J. Orloff (eds.), "Handbook of Renal Physiology," sec. 8, American Physiological Society, Wash., D.C., 1973.

Levinsky, N. G., and M. Levy: Clearance Techniques, in R. W. Berliner and J. Orloff (eds.), "Handbook of Renal Physiology," sec. 8, American Physiological Society, Wash., D.C., 1973.

Malvin, R. L., and W. S. Wilde: Stop-flow Technique, in R. W. Berliner and J. Orloff (eds.), "Handbook of Renal Physiology," sec. 8, American Physiological Society, Wash., D.C., 1973.

ANALYSIS OF INDIVIDUAL NEPHRON SEGMENTS

Chaps. 6 to 10 concern the renal handling of specific substances. Another organizational approach to renal physiology is to look at a particular nephron segment and describe the various transport characteristics of that segment. The Suggested Readings in this section, based largely on isolated-perfused-tubule work, follow this latter pattern.

Berry, C. A.: Heterogeneity of Tubular Transport Processes in the Nephron, *Ann. Rev. Physiol.,* **44**:181 (1982).

Jacobson, H. R.: Functional Segmentation of the Mammalian Nephron, *Am. J. Physiol.,* **241**:F205 (1981).

Jameson, R. L., H. Sonnenberg, and J. A. Stein: Questions and Replies: Role of the Collecting Tubule in Fluid, Sodium, and Potassium Balance, *Am. J. Physiol.,* **237**:F247 (1979).

Koeppen, B. M., B. A. Biagi, and G. Giebisch: Electrophysiology of Mammalian Renal Tubules, *Ann. Rev. Physiol.,* **45**:483 (1983).

Walker, L. A. and H. Valtin: Biological Importance of Nephron Heterogeneity, *Ann. Rev. Physiol.,* **44**:203 (1982).

Transport Characteristics of Nephron Segments (A Symposium), *Kidney Int.,* **22**:425 (1982).

CHAP. 1

Barajas, L.: Anatomy of the Juxtaglomerular Apparatus, *Am. J. Physiol.,* **237**:F333 (1979).

Beeuwkes, R., III: The Vascular Organization of the Kidney, *Ann. Rev. Physiol.,* **42**:531 (1980).

Beeuwkes, R., and J. V. Boventre: Tubular Organization and Vascular-tubular Relations in the Dog Kidney, *Am. J. Physiol.,* **229**:695 (1975). Read this to see how complex the anatomy really is.

Bulger, R. E., and D. C. Dobyan: Recent Advances in Renal Morphology, *Ann. Rev. Physiol.,* **44**:147 (1982).

Carretero, O. A., and A. G. Scicli: The Renal Kallikrein-kinin System, *Am. J. Physiol.,* **238**:F247 (1980).

Dunn, M. J.: Renal Prostaglandins, in S. Klahr and S. G. Massry (eds.), "Contemporary Nephrology, Vol. 1," Plenum, New York, 1981.

CHAP. 2

Aronson, P. S.: Identifying Secondary Active Solute Transport in Epithelia, *Am. J. Physiol.,* **240**:F1 (1981).

Brenner, B. M., and T. H. Hostetter: Molecular Basis of Proteinuria of Glomerular Origin, *N. Engl. J. Med.,* **298**:826(1978).

Brenner, B. M., and H. D. Humes: Mechanics of Glomerular Ultrafiltration, *N. Engl. J. Med.,* **297**:148 (1977).

Deen, W. M., C. R. Robertson, and B. M. Brenner: Glomerular Ultrafiltration, *Fed. Proc.,* **33**:14 (1974). The most concise review of glomerular pressures and the dependence of GFR on RBF.

Hayes, R. M.: Principles of Ion and Water Transport in the Kidney, *Hosp. Pract.,* Sept. (1978).

Hopfer, U.: Transport in Isolated Plasma Membranes, *Am. J. Physiol.,* **234**:F89 (1978).

Kassirer, J. P.: Clinical Evaluation of Kidney Function–Tubular Function, *N. Engl. J. Med.,* **285**:499 (1971).

Oken, D. E.: An Analysis of Glomerular Dynamics in Rat, Dog, and Man, *Kidney Int.,* **22**:136 (1982).

Pappenheimer, J. R.: Passage of Molecules through Capillary Walls, *Physiol. Rev.,* **33**:387 (1953). A discussion of the basic concepts and principles of ultrafiltration.

Schafer, J. A.: Membrane Transport, in S. Klahr and S. G. Massry (eds.), "Contemporary Nephrology, Vol. 1," Plenum, New York, 1981.

CHAP. 3

Kassirer, J. P.: Clinical Evaluation of Kidney Function—Glomerular Function, *N. Engl. J. Med.*, **285**:385 (1971).

Levinsky, N. G., and M. Levy: Clearance Techniques, in R. W. Berliner and J. Orloff (eds.), "Handbook of Renal Physiology," sec. 8, American Physiological Society, Wash., D.C., 1973.

Smith, H. W.: "Principles of Renal Physiology," chaps. 3–6, Oxford, New York, 1956.

Ganong, W. F.: The Brain Renin-angiotensin System, *Ann. Rev. Physiol.*, **46**:17 (1984).

Kriz, W.: Structural Organization of the Renal Medulla, *Am. J. Physiol.*, **241**:R3 (1981).

Margolius, H. S.: The Kallikrein-kinin System and the Kidney, *Ann. Rev. Physiol.*, **46**:309 (1984).

Nasjletti, A., and K. U. Malik: The Renal Kallikrein-kinin and Prostaglandin Systems Interactions, *Ann. Rev. Physiol.*, **81**:597 (1981).

Oliver, J.: "Nephrons and Kidneys: A Quantitative Study of Developmental and Evolutionary Mammalian Architectonics," Harper & Row, New York, 1968.

Peach, M. J.: Renin-angiotensin System: Biochemistry and Mechanisms of Action, *Physiol. Rev.*, **57**:313 (1977).

Prostaglandins and the Kidney (A Symposium), *Kidney Int.*, **19**:755–880 (1981).

Rouiller, C., and A. F. Muller (eds.): "The Kidney," vol. 1, Academic, New York, 1969.

Stein, J.: Hormones and the Kidney, *Hosp. Pract.*, July (1979).

Tisher, C. C.: Anatomy of the Kidney, in B. M. Brenner and F. C. Rector (eds.), "The Kidney," W. B. Saunders, Phila., 1981.

CHAP. 4

Burg, M. B.: The Nephron in Transport of Sodium, Amino Acids, and Glucose, *Hosp. Pract.*, Oct. (1978).

Carone, F. A., and D. R. Peterson: Hydrolysis and Transport of Small Peptides by the Proximal Tubule, *Am. J. Physiol.*, **238**:F151, 1980.

Grantham, J. J.: Studies of Organic Anion and Cation Transport in Isolated Segments of Proximal Tubules, *Kidney Int.*, **22**:514 (1982).

Gregor, R., F. Lang, and S. Silbernagl: "Renal Transport of Organic Substances," Springer-Verlag, New York, 1981. Contains excellent reviews of individual substances (PAH, uric acid, etc.)

Maunsbach, A. B.: Cellular Mechanisms of Tubular Protein Transport, in "Kidney and Urinary Tract Physiology II, International Review of Physiology, vol. II," University Park Press, Baltimore, 1976.

Rennick, B. R.: Renal Tubule Transport of Organic Cations, *Am. J. Physiol.*, **240**:F83 (1981).

Schafer, J. A., and D. W. Barfuss: Membrane Mechanisms for Transepithelial Amino Acid Absorption and Secretion, *Am. J. Physiol.*, **238**:F335 (1980).

CHAP. 5

Atlas, S. A., A. P. Niarchos, and D. B. Case: Inhibitors of the Renin-angiotensin System, *Am. J. Nephrol.*, **3**:118 (1983).

Aukland, K.: Methods for Measuring Renal Blood Flow: Total Flow and Regional Distribution, *Ann. Rev. Physiol.*, **42**:543 (1980).

Barger, A. A., and J. A. Herd: Renal Vascular Anatomy and Distribution of Blood Flow, in R. W. Berliner and J. Orloff (eds.), "Handbook of Renal Physiology," sec. 8, American Physiological Society, Wash., D.C., 1973.

Brenner, B. M. (ed.): Control of Glomerular Function by Intrinsic Contractile Elements (A Symposium), *Fed. Proc.*, **42**:3045 (1983).

Carretero, O. A., and A. G. Scicli: The Renal Kallikrein-kinin System, *Am. J. Physiol.*, **238**:F247 (1980).

Davis, J. O.: The Control of Renin Release, *Am. J. Med.*, **55**:333 (1973).

Dunn, M. J.: Renal Prostaglandins, in S. Klahr and S. G. Massry (eds.), "Contemporary Nephrology, Vol. 1," Plenum, New York, 1981.

Dworkin, L. D., I. Ilkuni, and B. M. Brenner: Hormonal Modulation of Glomerular Function, *Ann. J. Physiol.*, **244**:F95 (1983).

Henrich, W. L.: Role of Prostaglandins in Renin Secretion, *Kidney Int.*, **19**:822 (1981).

Insel, P. A., and M. D. Snavely: Catecholamines and the Kidney: Receptors and Renal Functions, *Ann. Rev. Physiol.*, **81**:625 (1981).

The Juxtaglomerular Apparatus (A Symposium), *Kidney Int.*, 22:S1–S220 (1982).

Kieton, T. K., and W. B. Campbell: The Pharmacologic Alteration of Renin Release, *Pharm. Rev.*, **32**:81 (1980).

Lee, M. R.: Dopamine and the Kidney, *Clin. Sci.*, **62**:439 (1982).

Levens, N. R., M. J. Peach, and R. M. Carey: Role of the Intrarenal Renin-angiotensin System in the Control of Renal Function, *Circ. Res.*, **48**:158 (1981).

Margolis, H.: The Kallikrein-kinin System and the Kidney, *Ann. Rev. Physiol.*, **46**:309 (1984).

Schnermann, J., and J. P. Briggs: Participation of Renal Cortical Prostaglandins in the Regulation of Glomerular Filtration Rate, *Kidney Int.*, **19**:802 (1981).

Spielman, W. S., and C. I. Thompson: A Proposed Role for Adenosine in the Regulation of Renal Hemodynamics and Renin Release, *Am. J. Physiol.*, **242**:F243 (1982).

Wright, F. S. (ed.): Feedback Control of Glomerular Filtration Rate (A Symposium), *Fed. Proc.*, **40**:77 (1981).

Wright, F. S., and J. P. Briggs: Feedback Control of Glomerular Blood Flow, Pressure, and Filtration Rate, *Physiol. Rev.*, **59**:958 (1979).

CHAP. 6

Andreoli, T. E., R. W. Berliner, J. P. Kokko, and D. J. Marsh: Questions and Replies: Renal Mechanisms for Urinary Concentrating and Diluting Processes, *Am. J. Physiol.,* **235**:F1 (1978).

Andreoli, T. E., and J. A. Schafer: Effective Luminal Hypotonicity: The Driving Force for Isotonic Proximal Tubular Fluid Absorption, *Am. J. Physiol.,* **236**:F89 (1979).

Berliner, R. W.: Mechanisms of Urine Concentration, *Kidney Int.,* **22**:2–8 (1982).

Berry, C. A.: Water Permeability Pathways in the Proximal Tubule, *Am. J. Physiol.,* **245**:F279 (1983).

Burg, M., and D. Good: Sodium Chloride Coupled Transport in Mammalian Nephrons, *Ann. Rev. Physiol.,* **45**:533 (1983).

Dousa, T. P.: Cellular Actions of Antidiuretic Hormone, *Min. Elect. Met.,* **5**:144 (1981).

Gross, P. A., R. W. Schrier, and R. J. Anderson: Prostaglandins and Water Metabolism, *Kidney Int.,* **19**:839 (1981).

Handler, J. S., and J. Orloff: Antidiuretic Hormone, *Ann. Rev. Physiol.,* **81**:611 (1981).

Herbert, S. C., and T. E. Andreoli: Water Movement Across the Mammalian Cortical Collecting Duct, *Kidney Int.,* **22**:526 (1982).

Jacobson, H. R.: Functional Segmentation of the Mammalian Nephron, *Am. J. Physiol.,* **241**:F205 (1981).

Jorgensen, P. L.: Sodium and Potassium Ion Pumps in Kidney Tubules, *Physiol. Rev.,* **60**:864 (1980).

Katz, A. I.: Renal Na-K-ATPase: Its Role in Tubular Sodium and Potassium Transport, *Am. J. Physiol.,* **242**:F207 (1982).

Kenpper, M., and M. Burg: Organization of Nephron Function, *Am. J. Physiol.,* **244**:F579 (1983).

Kokko, J. P.: Membrane Characteristics Governing Salt and Water Transport in the Loop of Henle, *Fed. Proc.,* **33**:25 (1974).

Kramer, H. J., K. Glanzer, and R. Dusing: Role of Prostaglandins in the Regulation of Renal Water Excretion, *Kidney Int.,* **19**:851 (1981).

Macknight, A. D. C., D. R. DiBona, and A. Leaf: Sodium Transport Across Toad Urinary Bladder: A Model "Tight" Epithelium, *Physiol. Rev.,* **60**:615 (1980).

Rector, F. C., Jr.: Sodium, Bicarbonate, and Chloride Absorption by the Proximal Tubule, *Am. J. Physiol.,* **244**:F461 (1983).

Schafer, J. A.: Salt and Water Absorption in the Proximal Tubule, *Physiologist,* **25**:95 (1982).

Schafer, J. A. (ed.): Water Transport in Epithelia (A Symposium), *Fed. Proc.,* **38**:120 (1979).

Schrier, R. W., and L. S. Linas: Mechanism of the Defect in Water Excretion in Adrenal Insufficiency, *Min. Elect. Met.,* **4**:1 (1980).

Stephenson, J. L. (ed.): Renal Concentrating Mechanism, *Fed. Proc.,* **42**:2377 (1983).

Stokes, J. B.: Integrated Actions of Renal Medullary Prostaglandins in the Control of Water Excretion, *Am. J. Physiol.,* **240**:F471 (1980).

Warnock, D. G., and J. Eveloff: NaCl Entry Mechanisms in the Luminal Membrane of the Renal Tubule, *Am. J. Physiol.*, **242**:F561 (1982).

See also articles under "Analysis of Individual Nephron Segments."

CHAP. 7

Anderson, B.: Regulation of Water Intake, *Physiol. Rev.*, **58**:582 (1978).

Atlas, S. A., A. P. Niarchos, and D. B. Case: Inhibitors of the Renin-angiotensin System, *Am. J. Nephrol.*, **3**:118 (1983).

Bie, P.: Osmoreceptors, Vasopressin, and Control of Renal Water Excretion, *Physiol. Rev.*, **60**:961 (1980).

Buckalew, V. J., Jr., and K. A. Gruber: Natriuretic Hormone, *Ann. Rev. Physiol.*, **46**:343 (1984).

Cannon, P. J.: The Kidney in Heart Failure, *N. Engl. J. Med.*, **296**:26 (1977).

Cowley, A. W., Jr., E. W. Quillen, Jr., and M. M. Skelton: Role of Vasopressin in Cardiovascular Regulation, *Fed. Proc.*, **42**:3170 (1983).

Davis, J. O.: The Control of Renin Release, *Am. J. Med.*, **55**:333 (1973).

Denton, D. A.: Salt Appetite, in C. F. Code and W. Heidel (eds.), "Handbook of Physiology," sec. 6, vol. I, American Physiological Society, Wash., D.C., 1967.

De Wardener, H. E.: The Control of Sodium Excretion, *Am. J. Physiol.*, **235**:F163 (1978).

De Wardener, H. E., and E. M. Clarkson, The Natriuretic Hormone: Recent Developments, *Clin. Sci.*, **63**:415 (1982).

DiBona, G. F.: Neural Control of Renal Tubular Sodium Reabsorption in the Dog, *Fed. Proc.*, **37**:1214 (1978).

Dunn, M. J.: Renal Prostaglandins, in S. Klahr and S. G. Massry (eds.), "Contemporary Nephrology, Vol. 1," Plenum, New York, 1981.

Earley, L. E., and R. W. Schrier: Intrarenal Control of Sodium Excretion by Hemodynamic and Physical Factors, in R. W. Berliner and J. Orloff (eds.), "Handbook of Renal Physiology," sec. 8, American Physiological Society, Wash., D.C., 1973.

Fanestil, D., and C. S. Park: Steroid Hormones and the Kidney, *Ann. Rev. Physiol.*, **81**:637 (1981).

Gauer, D. H., and J. P. Henry: Circulatory Basis of Fluid Volume Control, *Physiol. Rev.*, **43**:423 (1963).

Häberle, D. A., and H. von Baeyer: Characteristics of Glomerulotubular Balance, *Am. J. Physiol.*, **244**:F355 (1983).

Insel, P. A., and M. D. Snavely: Catecholamines and the Kidney: Receptors and Renal Function, *Ann. Rev. Physiol.*, **81**:625 (1981).

Jacobson, H. R., and D. W. Seldin: Proximal Tubular Reabsorption and Its Regulation, *Ann. Rev. Pharm. Toxicol.*, **17**:623 (1977).

Knox, F. G., et al.: Escape from the Sodium-retaining Effects of Mineralocorticoids, *Kidney Int.*, **17**:263 (1980).

Kokko, J. P.: Effects of Prostaglandins on Renal Epithelial Electrolyte Transport, *Kidney Int.*, **19**:791 (1981).

Laragh, J. H., and J. E. Sealey: The Renin-angiotensin-aldosterone Hormonal System and Regulation of Sodium, Potassium, and Blood Pressure Homeostasis, in R. W. Berliner and J. Orloff (eds.), "Handbook of Renal Physiology," sec. 8, American Physiological Society, Wash., D.C., 1973.

Lote, C. J.: Renal Prostaglandins and Sodium Excretion, *Quart. J. Exp. Physiol.,* **67**:377 (1982).

Marver, D.: Evidence of Corticosteroid Action Along the Nephron, *Am. J. Physiol.,* **246**:F111 (1984).

Mills, I. H.: The Renal Kallikrein-kinin System and Sodium Excretion, *Quart. J. Exp. Physiol.,* **67**:393 (1982).

Reid, I. A., B. J. Morris, and W. F. Ganong: The Renin-angiotensin System, *Ann. Rev. Physiol.,* **40**:377 (1978).

Robertson, G. L., R. L. Shelton, and S. Atkar: The Osmoregulation of Vasopressin, *Kidney Int.,* **10**:25 (1976).

Sawchenko, P. E., and M. I. Friedman: Sensory Functions of the Liver — A Review, *Am. J. Physiol.,* **236**:R5 (1979).

Schrier, R. W., and T. Berl: Nonosmolar Factors Affecting Renal Water Excretion, *N. Engl. J. Med.,* **292**:81 (1975).

Schrier, R. W., T. Berl, and R. J. Anderson: Osmotic and Nonosmotic Control of Vasopressin Release, *Am. J. Physiol.,* **236**:F321 (1979).

Smith, H. W.: Salt and Water Volume Receptors, *Am. J. Med.,* **23**:623 (1957).

Stokes, J. B.: Integrated Actions of Renal Medullary Prostaglandins in the Control of Water Excretion, *Am. J. Physiol.,* **240**:F471 (1981).

Weingartner, H., et al.: Effects of Vasopressin on Human Memory Functions, *Science,* **211**:601 (1981).

Windhager, E. E.: Some Aspects of Proximal Tubular Salt Reabsorption, *Fed. Proc.,* **33**:21 (1974).

CHAP. 8

Adrogue, H. J., and N. E. Madias: Changes in Plasma Potassium Concentration during Acute Acid-base Disturbances, *Am. J. Med.,* **71**:456 (1981).

Bia, M. J., and R. A. De Fronzo: Extrarenal Potassium Homeostasis, *Am. J. Physiol.,* **240**:F257 (1981).

Gennari, F. J., and J. J. Cohen: Role of the Kidney in Potassium Homeostasis: Lessons from Acid-base Disturbances, *Kidney Int.,* **8**:1 (1975). Attempts to explain the mechanisms by which potassium excretion is influenced by acid-base disturbances.

Giebisch, G., and B. Stanton: Potassium Transport in the Nephron, *Ann. Rev. Physiol.,* **41**:241 (1979).

Hayslett, J. P., and H. J. Binder: Mechanism of Potassium Adaptation, *Am. J. Physiol.,* **243**:F103 (1982).

Jacobson, H. R.: Functional Segmentation of the Mammalian Nephron, *Am. J. Physiol.,* **241**:F205 (1981).

Jamison, R. L., J. Work, and J. A. Schafer: New Pathways for Potassium Transport in the Kidney, *Am. J. Physiol.,* **242**:F297 (1982).

Jorgensen, P. L.: Sodium and Potassium Ion Pumps in Kidney Tubules, *Physiol. Rev.,* **60**:864 (1980).

Katz, A. I.: Renal Na-K-ATPase: Its Role in Tubular Sodium and Potassium Transport, *Am. J. Physiol.,* **242**:F207 (1982).

Knochel, J. P.: Role of Glucoregulatory Hormones in Potassium Homeostasis, *Kidney Int.,* **11**:443 (1977).

Stanton, B. A., and G. H. Giebisch: Regulation of Potassium Homeostasis, in R. A. Corradino (ed.), "Functional Regulation at the Cellular and Molecular Level," Elsevier, New York, 1982.

Stearns, R. H., et al.: Internal Potassium Balance and the Control of the Plasma Potassium Concentration, *Medicine,* **60**:339 (1981).

Wright, F. S.: Sites and Mechanisms of Potassium Transport along the Renal Tubule, *Kidney Int.,* **11**:415 (1977).

Wright, F. S., and G. Giebisch: Renal Potassium Transport: Contributions of Different Nephron Segments and Populations, *Am. J. Physiol.,* **235**:F515 (1978).

See also articles listed under "Analysis of Individual Nephron Segments."

CHAP. 9

Aronson, P. S.: Mechanisms of Active H^+ Secretion in the Proximal Tubule, *Am. J. Physiol.,* **245**:F647 (1983).

Arruda, J. A. L., and N. A. Kurtzman: Relationship of Renal Sodium and Water Transport to Hydrogen Ion Secretion, *Ann. Rev. Physiol.,* **40**:43 (1978).

Arruda, J. A. L., and N. A. Kurtzman: Mechanisms and Classification of Deranged Distal Urinary Acidification, *Am. J. Phsiol.,* **239**:F515 (1980).

Berry, C. A., and D. C. Warnock: Acidification in the In Vitro Perfused Tubule, *Kidney Int.,* **22**:507 (1982).

Dobyan, D. C., and R. E. Bulger: Renal Carbonic Anhydrase, *Am. J. Physiol.,* **243**:F311 (1982).

Jacobson, H. R., and D. W. Seldin: On the Generation, Maintenance, and Correction of Metabolic Alkalosis, *Am. J. Physiol.,* **245**:F425 (1983).

Kurtzman, N. A., and J. A. L. Arruda: Physiologic Significance of Urinary Carbon Dioxide Tension, *Min. Elect. Met.,* **1**:241 (1978).

Madias, N. E., H. J. Androgue, and J. J. Cohen: Maladaptive Renal Response to Secondary Hypercapnia in Chronic Metabolic Alkalosis, *Am. J. Physiol.,* **238**:F283 (1980).

Malnic, G.: Cellular Mechanisms of Urinary Acidification, *Min. Elect. Met.,* **5**:66 (1981).

Maren, T. B.: Chemistry of the Renal Reabsorption of Bicarbonate, *Can. J. Biochem. Physiol.,* **52**:1041 (1974).

Rector, F. C., Jr.: Sodium, Bicarbonate, and Chloride Reabsorption by the Proximal Tubule, *Am. J. Physiol.,* **244**:F461 (1983).

Rector, F. C., Jr.: Acidification of the Urine, in R. W. Berliner and J. Orloff (eds.), "Handbook of Renal Physiology," sec. 8, American Physiological Society, Wash., D.C., 1973.

Schwartz, W. B., C. Van Ypersele de Strihou, and J. P. Kassirer: Role of Anions in Metabolic Alkalosis and Potassium Deficiency, *N. Engl. J. Med.*, **279**:630 (1968).

Seldin, D. W., and F. C. Rector, Jr.: The Generation and Maintenance of Metabolic Alkalosis, *Kidney Int.*, **1**:306 (1972).

Steinmetz, P. R.: Cellular Mechanisms of Urinary Acidification, *Physiol. Rev.*, **54**:890(1974).

Tannen, R. L.: Ammonia Metabolism, *Am. J. Physiol.*, **235**:F265(1978).

See also articles listed under "Analysis of Individual Nephron Segments."

CHAP. 10

Agus, Z. S., S. Goldfarb, and A. Wasserstein: Mineral Metabolism in Health and Disease, in S. Klahr and S. G. Massry (eds.), "Contemporary Nephrology, Vol. 1," Plenum, New York, 1981.

Austin, L. A., and H. Heath, III: Calcitonin: Physiology and Pathophysiology, *N. Engl. J. Med.*, **304**:269 (1981).

DeLucca, H. F.: The Kidney as an Endocrine Organ for the Production of 1,25-dihydroxyvitamin D_3, a Calcium-mobilizing Hormone, *N. Engl. J. Med.*, **289**:359 (1973).

Dennis, V. W., and P. C. Brazy: Divalent Anion Transport in Isolated Renal Tubules, *Kidney Int.*, **22**:498 (1982).

Fraser, D. R.: Regulation of the Metabolism of Vitamin D, *Physiol. Rev.*, **60**:550 (1980).

Lang, F., R. Greger, F. G. Knox, and H. Oberleithner: Factors Modulating the Renal Handling of Phosphate, *Renal Physiol.*, **4**:1 (1981).

Lemann, J., Jr., N. D. Adams, and R. W. Gray: Urinary Calcium Excretion in Human Beings, *N. Engl. J. Med.*, **301**:535 (1979).

Massry, S. G., and J. W. Coburn: The Hormonal and Non-hormonal Control of Renal Excretion of Calcium and Magnesium, *Nephron,* **10**:66 (1973).

Ng, R. C. K., R. A. Peraino, and W. N. Suki: Divalent Cation Transport in Isolated Tubules. *Kidney Int.*, **22**:492 (1982).

Quamme, G. A., and J. H. Dirks: Magnesium Transport in the Nephron, *Am. J. Physiol.*, **239**:F393 (1980).

Suki, W. N.: Calcium Transport in the Nephron, *Am. J. Physiol.*, **237**:F1 (1979).

Suki, W. N., and D. Rouse: Mechanisms of Calcium Transport, *Min. Elect. Met.*, **5**:175 (1981).

See also articles listed under "Analysis of Individual Nephron Segments."

STAYING UP-TO-DATE

The most painless way for a busy clinician not specializing in nephrology to follow important developments in renal physiology is to read the excellent reviews which appear frequently in the *New England Journal of Medicine* and *Hospital Practice*. They are usually succinct and emphasize the clinical implications of new research findings. More detailed reviews are to be found in the Annual Review of Physiology and in the specialty journals for renal physiology, notably the *American Journal of Physiology* (Renal and Electrolyte Section), *Kidney International*, *Renal Physiology*, and *Mineral and Electrolyte Metabolism*. The journals *Hypertension* and *Circulation Research* frequently have reviews on the renin-angiotensin system.

INDEX